Critical Care Nutrition
Therapy for Non-nutritionists

W0112556

Mette M. Berger
Editor

Critical Care Nutrition Therapy for Non-nutritionists

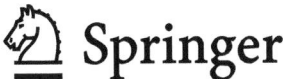 Springer

Editor
Mette M. Berger
Service of Intensive Care
Medicine and Burns
Lausanne University Hospital
(CHUV)
Lausanne
Switzerland

ISBN 978-3-319-58651-9   ISBN 978-3-319-58652-6   (eBook)
https://doi.org/10.1007/978-3-319-58652-6

Library of Congress Control Number: 2017962014

Printed on acid-free paper

This Springer imprint is published by Springer Nature
The registered company is Springer International Publishing AG
The registered company address is: Gewerbestrasse 11, 6330 Cham, Switzerland

Foreword

The essentials, not a complete catalog of the existing knowledge!

This book is about metabolic and nutrition support during critical illness. It summarizes the up-to-date and vital knowledge to optimize the nutrition care for most of the critically ill patients. As a result, the described knowledge required for routine care is easy to access for nonexperts in nutrition. It is not one more book for intensive care physicians; it is the pocket book that allows to retrieve the needed information in order to take the right decision in due time.

Physicians are overwhelmed by the massive amount of information. Scientific journals mostly present the results of great prospective trials, meta-analysis of very heterogeneous patient populations, and case reports of rare situations. Scholar reviews in prestigious journals, written by experts, show sophisticated views on narrow questions. Most of these papers suffer from the absence of summary specifying the to-do list for the medical decisions at the bedside of patient. There is no doubt that scientific journals greatly contribute to level up the medical knowledge and certainly stimulate advances in basic and clinical research. Unfortunately, the conclusions of the published papers are often difficult to use in daily practice. In addition, a number of these conclusions are controversial, as they are generated by cutting-edge clinical research either on specific conditions or sophisticated modalities not yet implemented in routine care in most institutions.

The relevant question is therefore: How good are the decisions and the prescriptions made by a physician unable to find the relevant information in the daily clinical rushing? A straightforward answer is "Rather poor, or unhealthy!"

To solve this dilemma and help physicians surviving the intensive care environment (!), the book carefully avoids diluting the most relevant knowledge into a complete description of all the existing pathologies. In other words, it summarizes the *essentials*. International experts have summarized their knowledge in brief chapters, palatable for nonexperts in nutrition. Practical recommendations are presented for common situations. Whenever different recommendations are possible, as a result of inconclusive study results, pragmatic recommendations are proposed. Their clinical validity is secured by a peer-review process to avoid (too) biased statements.

Professor MM Berger is one of the lead physicians in the field of nutrition and metabolism. She has designed and edited this book. I am greatly thankful to her for this tremendous effort. You are likely to share my views, once you have used the book. Your patients are likely not to ever see this book, but they will benefit from you for having used it!

Claude Pichard, M.D., Ph.D.

Contents

Contributors

Itai Bendavid Department of General Intensive Care and Institute for Nutrition Research, Rabin Medical Center, Beilinson Hospital, Petah Tikva, Israel

Sackler School of Medicine, Tel Aviv University, Tel Aviv, Israel

Mette M. Berger, M.D., Ph.D. Service of Intensive Care Medicine and Burns, Lausanne University Hospital (CHUV), Lausanne, Switzerland

Luisa Bonafé, M.D. Division of Genetic Medicine, Center for Molecular Diseases, Lausanne University Hospital, Lausanne, Switzerland

Lionel Bouvet, M.D. Department of Anesthesia and Intensive Care, Hospice Civils Lyon, Lyon, France

Mélanie Charrière, R.D. Service of Intensive Care Medicine and Burns, Nutrition Clinique, Lausanne University Hospital (CHUV), Lausanne, Switzerland

Jean-Michel Constantin, M.D Department of Perioperative Medicine, University Hospital of Clermont-Ferrand, Clermont-Ferrand, France

David C. Frankenfield, M.S., R.D. Department of Clinical Nutrition, Department of Nursing, Penn State Health System, Milton S. Hershey Medical Center, Pennsylvania, USA

Carole Ichai, M.D., Ph.D. University Hospital of Nice, Intensive Care Unit, Pasteur 2 Hospital, Nice, France

Jeffrey I. Mechanick, M.D. The Marie-Josee and Henry R. Kravis Center for Cardiovascular Health at Mount Sinai Heart, New York, NY, USA

Divisions of Cardiology and Endocrinology, Diabetes and Bone Disease, Icahn School of Medicine at Mount Sinai, New York, NY, USA

Michael C. Müller Department of Anesthesiology and Operative Intensive Care Medicine, Charité—Universitätsmedizin Berlin, Campus Virchow-Klinikum, Berlin, Germany

Heleen M. Oudemans-van Straaten, M.D. Department of Intensive Care, VU University Medical Center, Amsterdam, The Netherlands

Olivier Pantet, M.D. Service of Adult Intensive Care Medicine and Burns, Lausanne University Hospital (CHUV), Lausanne, Switzerland

Sébastien Perbet, M.D. Department of Perioperative Medicine, University Hospital of Clermont-Ferrand, Clermont-Ferrand, France

Hervé Quintard, M.D., Ph.D. Intensive Care Unit, Pasteur 2 Hospital, Nice, France

Annika Reintam-Blaser, M.D. Intensive Care, Lucerne Cantonal Hospital, Lucerne, Switzerland

University of Tartu, Tartu, Estonia

Antoine Schneider, **M.D., Ph.D.** Service de Médecine Intensive Adulte et Centre de Brûlés, Centre Hospitalier et Universitaire Vaudois (CHUV), Lausanne, Switzerland

Pierre Singer Department of General Intensive Care and Institute for Nutrition Research, Rabin Medical Center, Beilinson Hospital, Petah Tikva, Israel

Sackler School of Medicine, Tel Aviv University, Tel Aviv, Israel

Luboš Sobotka, M.D. Department of Medicine, Metabolic Care and Gerontology, Medical Faculty Hradec Kralove, Charles University in Prague, Hradec Kralove, Czech Republic

Christel Tran Division of Genetic Medicine, Center for Molecular Diseases, Lausanne University Hospital, Lausanne, Switzerland

Michael A. Via, M.D. Division of Endocrinology, Diabetes, and Bone Disease, Mount Sinai Beth Israel Medical Center, Icahn School of Medicine at Mount Sinai, New York, NY, USA

Steffen Weber-Carstens, M.D. Department of Anesthesiology and Operative Intensive Care Medicine, Charité— Universitätsmedizin Berlin, Campus Virchow-Klinikum, Berlin, Germany

Berlin Institute of Health (BIH), Berlin, Germany

Tobias Wollersheim, M.D. Department of Anesthesiology and Operative Intensive Care Medicine, Charité— Universitätsmedizin Berlin, Campus Virchow-Klinikum, Berlin, Germany

Berlin Institute of Health (BIH), Berlin, Germany

Chapter 1
General ICU Patients

Mette M. Berger

This pocket book is dedicated to the intensive care physicians who take care of the critically ill patients on a daily basis. Nowadays, most doctors are bewildered by the controversies that increase the uncertainty as to the optimal metabolic management of their patients. Orientation becomes even more important with the appearance of a new category of intensive care (ICU) patients, the chronic critically ill (CCI). This book attempts to provide a rational, physiology-based way to deal with the most common questions while signalling areas of controversy [1].

This first chapter will address the generalities such as criteria to identify the patients in need of artificial nutrition, defining their basic needs, the timing of an intervention and the general monitoring tools. Specific organ failures, as well as related needs and the caveats, will be addressed in the following chapters.

M.M. Berger
Service of Intensive Care Medicine and Burns,
Lausanne University Hospital (CHUV), Lausanne, Switzerland
e-mail: mette.berger@chuv.ch

© Springer International Publishing AG 2018   1
M.M. Berger (ed.), *Critical Care Nutrition Therapy
for Non-nutritionists*, https://doi.org/10.1007/978-3-319-58652-6_1

1.1 Definition of the Critical Care Patient

What defines critical illness? The patients are admitted to an ICU because of organ failure due to an overwhelming infection, trauma or other types of tissue injury that render them dependent on complex mechanical and pharmacological therapies. They present an intense inflammatory response, which is a coordinated cytokine-, hormone- and nervous system-mediated series of events that alter temperature regulation and energy expenditure. This in turn invokes neuroendocrine and hematologic responses, reorients the synthesis and disposition of several proteins in the body and dramatically stimulates muscle protein catabolism [2]. The resulting catabolic critical illness is a life-threatening condition that complicates the admission condition and further compromises quality of life and outcome.

Which are the criteria enabling the identification of the patients with an indication to a nutritional intervention? The "bed and breakfast patients", i.e. those staying up to 72 h in the ICU and resume oral feeding rather easily, are obviously not the target population. Figure 1.1 provides some criteria that can assist selecting the patients in need of metabolic therapy.

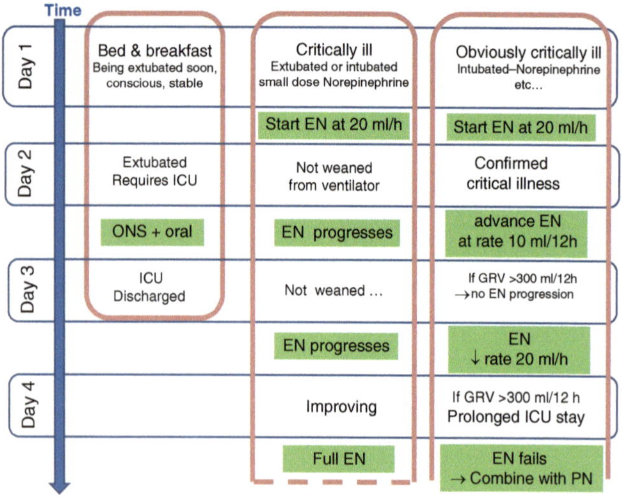

FIGURE 1.1 Categories of patients and potential nutritional management (*GRV* gastric residual volume, *ONS* oral nutrition supplement)

Table 1.1 Scores assisting the identification of patients at metabolic risk

Score	Equation	Comments
NRS 2002 Nutrition risk screening score	(A) (BMI, weight loss, and food intake) (0–3 points each); (B) (severity of disease 0–3); (C) age (>70 years = 1 point) NRS = worst A+ B + C; maximum 7 points	1 point in any of the A should be consider high risk, as ICU admission generates 3 points
MUST 2003 Malnutrition universal screening tool	BMI (0–2 points) + unplanned weight loss (0–2 points) + acute disease effect (2 points) Maximum MUST 6 points	0 point low risk; 1 = medium risk (observe); 2 high risk (treat)
NUTRIC modified (without IL-6)	Age (0–2 points), APACHE II score (0–3 points), SOFA score (0–2 points), number of comorbidities (0–1), days from hospital admission to ICU admission (0–1)	5–9 points: high risk 0–4: low risk

Scores will assist a more precise definition of patients at risk of nutritional problems. The European nutrition risk screening score (NRS) [3] and British MUST (Table 1.1) are the easiest to use although they have not been validated for ICU patients, being developed as screening tools for general hospital patients. Nevertheless, according to the upcoming ICU guidelines of the European Society for Clinical Nutrition (ESPEN) [4], the NRS remains the simplest and fastest tool. In the NRS, an ICU admission results in three risk points (out of seven maximum); therefore, a nutrition-related alteration is required to create a real metabolic risk, which is the reason why ESPEN recommends considering five points as the risk level prompting therapy (Fig. 1.2). The Canadian NUTRIC score was designed as a specific critical care score and is still

Preadmission food intake + Other risk factors	Normal feeding until ICU admission No risk factor NRS = 3(4)	No food intake for 3–4 days NRS = 5	No food intake for >4 days Malnutrition NRS>5
Intervention	Observe	Initiate EN within 48 hours of admission	Initiate EN or PN within first 48 hours of admission

FIGURE 1.2 Types of nutritional intervention based on screening criteria

not prospectively validated: its computing is dominated by the weight of two ICU severity scores (APACHE and SOFA scores), includes no nutrition criteria and takes more time to complete [5], reasons why ESPEN does not recommend it as screening tool.

Figure 1.2 proposes a strategy to integrate the anamnestic information and the NRS score to decide about a nutrition intervention.

1.2   Timing

For metabolic reasons, tree periods should be considered: (1) the early phase, i.e. the first 48 h, (2) the stabilization phase and (3) in some patients, the chronic-acute phase that starts after 2–3 weeks and may last for months and implies important changes in body composition. The majority of patients will leave the ICU by the end of the stabilization phase. Should we start feeding at a full regimen immediately?

There are two main reasons not to full feed immediately:

(a) The endogenous energy and glucose production, as per below
(b) The risk of inappropriate refeeding syndrome

Endogenous energy production: During the early phase in the absence of external supply (i.e. starvation), the body is able to produce glucose on its own for the glucose-depending

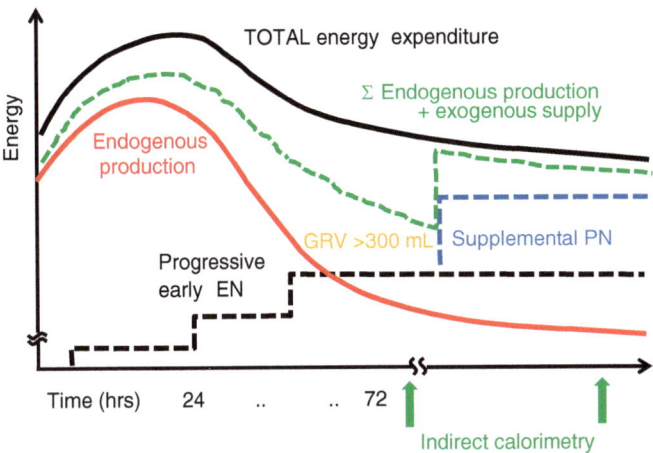

FIGURE 1.3 Conceptual presentation of optimal feeding strategy to avoid both overfeeding and underfeeding in critical illness (Reproduced with permission from Oshima et al. 2017 [6])

organs by glycolysis and endogenous glucose production already after 12 h of feeding interruption [6]. The endogenous production is maximal during the first 48 h then abates: the amounts produced can only be measured by tracer techniques that are not available in clinical settings. Therefore, whatever the route, the administration of feeds should follow a progressive pattern to respect this endogenous response (Fig. 1.3), and thereby prevent early overloading with extrinsic substrates at a period which is characterized by elevated insulin resistance.

Refeeding syndrome risk: During complete or partial starvation, evolutionary adaptation has conferred the organism the above protecting mechanisms. Some adaptations occur very rapidly (within hours) such as the reduction of the endogenous insulin secretion and the consequent changes in the fluxes of electrolytes. The next step of shut down is more complex and occurs around the third day of starvation with increased ketone body production in healthy subjects, but not in critically ill patients, who are facing an intense catabolism to deliver amino acids for continued endogenous glucose production. Any glucose supply will induce a nearly immediate reversal of this strategy and prompt insulin secretion as well as its consequences on electrolyte movements. The progressive reintroduction of feeds enables monitoring of this response and supplying the required phosphate, potassium and magnesium supplements, preventing devastating effects [7].

1.3   What Are the Needs?

How should we determine the individual patient's needs? What are the factors to consider? A frequently unsolved question is "what is the patient's weight"? The "preadmission weight" is often unknown, and the "actual weight" sometimes obtained in the ICU is frequently artificially increased by fluid resuscitation. The pragmatic solution is to use the preadmission weight if known and an observer's estimation of it in absence of such information.

As previously mentioned, it is essential to distinguish the very early phase (first 48 h) from the stabilization phase and the subacute-chronic phase which starts at around the end of the second week and may last for months.

Energy: This topic has generated major controversy. Multiple equations exist which have all been shown to be inexact compared to an indirect calorimetry, which is the gold standard [8, 9], but the latter equipment is not yet widely available. The least inexact equations are the Penn State University for ICU patients and the Toronto equation for major burns, both being derived from multiple indirect calorimetric determinations (Table 1.2). The simplest appreciation is to use 20 (first days) and 25 (stabilization) kcal/kg*day as target. A target guided by repeated indirect calorimetry will become the standard when upcoming simpler devices become available.

Proteins: The requirements should be dissociated from energy intakes, a differentiation which is difficult in clinical practice due to the fixed combinations of energy and proteins proposed by the industry. The World Health Organisation

TABLE 1.2 Most common energy target equations

Name	Equation
Harris and Benedict	M: REE = 66.47 + (13.75 × weight) + (5.0 × height) − (6.76 × age) F: REE = 655.1 + (9.56 × weight) + (1.85 × height) − (4.68 × age)
Penn State 2003	Total EE = (0.85 × REE-HB) + (175 × T_{max}) + (33 × V·E) − 6′433
Toronto equation	Total EE = −4343 + (10.5 × %BSA) + (0.23 × CI) + (0.84 × REE-HB) + (114 × T °C) − (4.5 × day after injury)
ESPEN 2009	Early phase: 20 kcal/kg*day to be achieved over 3 days
	Stable phase: 25 (or indirect calorimetry)

REE-HB Harris and Benedict estimation of resting energy expenditure, *CI* caloric intake, *T °C* temperature in Celsius, *V·E* minute volume (in L/min), height in cm, weight in kg

recommends 0.8 g/kg/day for healthy subjects. During the last decade, several studies have shown this amount to be insufficient for critically ill patients. The recommendations have been progressively increased to 1.3–1.5 g/kg*day [10]. Some categories of patients such as major burns have requirements as high as 2.0 g/kg*day based on isotopic studies (see Chap. 5): the elevated requirements of obese patients are discussed in Chap. 8 and those of renal failure patients in Chap. 9.

Carbohydrates: Several organs are strictly glucose dependent (brain, leukocytes) during the first 24 h of starvation, while others can adapt to a combination of substrates (heart, kidney, muscle, liver, adipose tissue). Too much glucose results in *de novo lipogenesis*, i.e. triglyceride synthesis at the liver level. The maximal tolerable glucose intake has been determined by tracer studies to be 5.0 mg/kg*min (i.e. 7.2 g/kg/day). Clinically, while 2.0 g/kg*day is the strict minimum requirement, doses of up to 4.0 g/kg*day cover needs without exposing the patient to overload.

Fat: Lipids are a necessary component of nutrition. In parenteral nutrition, the debate has been about the optimal combination of different types of fatty acids (n-3, n-9 and n-6 fatty acids) to achieve anti-inflammatory effects [11] and the total amount of lipids provided enterally and intravenously. In case of lipid-free parenteral nutrition (PN), essential fatty acid deficiency can be detected already after 5 days. Therefore lipids should be delivered with other substrates, the minimum daily amount being 0.5 g/kg*day to cover essential fatty acid needs, while an exact maximum has not been determined: the ESPEN guidelines recommend a total amount of fat not exceeding 1.5 g/kg*day.

Micronutrients: The requirements will depend on the severity of disease and route of feeding. While a dose corresponding to the recommended daily intake (RDI) is usually included in enteral feeds, this is by definition not the case with parenteral nutrition for stability reasons: micronutrients must be provided separately on a daily basis. The ESPEN guidelines underline the necessity to provide one daily dose of trace elements and vitamins for each day on PN [12]. Reinforcement of antioxidant defences with doses of micronutrients up to ten times the recommended PN has been associated with reduction of complications [13]. On the other hand, high-dose selenium monotherapy does not improve outcome [14].

1.4   Enteral and Parenteral Routes

The enteral route is to be preferred, whenever not contraindicated, for many non-nutritional reasons such as stimulation of gut immunity and maintenance of intestinal function. But in case of absolute contraindication (Table 1.3), the parenteral route is a valuable and safe alternative as shown by the most recent trials and meta-analysis [15]. Feeding by the enteral route should be initiated as early as possible to "prevent losing it", i.e. within 24–48 h. The 2017 guidelines of the ESICM expert group recommend early enteral feeding with only five exceptions where delay is recommended (relative

TABLE 1.3 Absolute contraindications to enteral feeding

Intestinal obstruction

Absence of intestinal continuity (temporary or definitive situation after surgical resection)

Acute intestinal ischaemia

Acute intestinal bleeding

contraindication): active gastric bleeding, overt bowel ischaemia, gastric residuals >500 mL, abdominal compartment syndrome and high output intestinal fistulae [16].

Using the gut is most successful when attempted within 24 h of admission and before the oedema from resuscitation affects the intestines and reduces their motility. This does however not mean that full feeding is to be achieved immediately (see Sect. 1.2).

Parenteral nutrition timing is still a matter of debate because of the negative results from studies carried in the 1980s and 1990s period, during which energy targets were much higher and glucose control nonexisting. Since the 2000, several large-size studies have been published showing that the outcome after PN compares to EN provided overfeeding is avoided [17]. Two recent large RCTs have shown equipoise between EN and PN when using early rapid progression to energy targets set by equations [18, 19]. Nevertheless, considering the potential non-nutritional benefits of EN and the higher costs of PN, its use should be limited to conditions where EN is contraindicated or insufficient to cover energy and protein needs.

1.5   Monitoring

Like any ICU therapy, the nutritional intervention should be monitored. Two aspects should be assessed: (1) what the patient really receives and (2) how the patient responds to the delivered nutrients (Fig. 1.4).

1. Feed delivery by the enteral route is frequently lower than 60% of prescription and should be closely monitored. It has

Variable	4*/day	Daily	2*/week	Weekly
Blood glucose	Daily	×		
Blood K, P, Mg	First day	×		
Insulin delivery (total per 24 h)		×		
Energy balance = E.target–E.delivery		×		Cumulated first week
Triglycerides			×	
ASAT, ALAT			×	
Prealbumin				×
Energy expenditure (indirect calorimetry)			Ideal	×
Weight (actual)		Major burns	Ideal	×
Stool emission			×	
Gastric residual vol.		Every 12 h first 3 days		

FIGURE 1.4 Proposed standard monitoring and timing of follow-up during the first week

repeatedly and worldwide been shown that delivery of nutrients is inferior (very rarely superior) to prescription, and the difference may be important enough to cause underfeeding [20]. Feeding to measured target whatever the route is not only clinically beneficial but also economically rewarding, as it reduces costly infectious complications [21]. The total protein delivery should be carefully watched as adequate provision contributes to reduce lean body mass loss.

2. The patient's response should be observed on a daily basis. Search for decreasing blood phosphate and potassium and changes in blood glucose during the first 48 hours of feeding is mandatory. The 24hr insulin requirements should be watched, followed after 3–4 days by liver tests and triglycerides. A daily clinical abdominal examination is mandatory as observation of stool frequency.

The patient's energy requirements change over time, generally in parallel with the decreasing lean body mass: repeated indirect calorimetry, at least once weekly, in long stayers is the only way to address the real requirements.

The patients staying for 7–10 days in the ICU while not intubated constitute a real problem with a high risk of underfeeding that will be addressed in Chap. 13. Only monitoring of real intakes (oral supplements, food) enables detection of a growing energy deficit.

1.6   Conclusion

The nutritional therapy of the critically ill can be initiated in a simple way with two recommendations: "try progressive enteral early and beware of refeeding syndrome". The 3 first days will be taken care of in most patients that way. The sicker patients will thereafter require more precise adjustments and monitoring.

References

1. Preiser JC, van Zanten ARH, Berger MM, Biolo G, Casaer M, Doig G, et al. Metabolic and nutritional support of critically ill patients: consensus and controversies. Crit Care. 2015;19:35.
2. Hoffer LJ, Bistrian BR. Nutrition in critical illness: a current conundrum. F1000Research. 2016;5:2531.
3. Kondrup J, Rasmussen HH, Hamberg O, Stanga Z. Nutritional risk screening (NRS 2002): a new method based on an analysis of controlled clinical trials. Clin Nutr. 2003;22:321–36.
4. Singer P, Reintam Blaser A, Berger MM, Calder P, Casear M, Hiesmayr M et al. ESPEN guidelines for the critically ill patient. Clin Nutr. 2018;38: in press.
5. Rahman A, Hasan RM, Agarwala R, Martin C, Day AG, Heyland DK. Identifying critically-ill patients who will benefit most from nutritional therapy: further validation of the "modified NUTRIC" nutritional risk assessment tool. Clin Nutr. 2016;35:158–62.

6. Oshima T, Berger MM, De Waele E, Guttormsen AB, Heidegger CP, Hiesmayr M, et al. Indirect calorimetry in nutritional therapy. A position paper by the ICALIC Study Group. Clin Nutr. 2017;36:651–62.

7. Doig GS, Simpson F, Heighes PT, Bellomo R, Chesher D, Caterson ID, et al. Restricted versus continued standard caloric intake during the management of refeeding syndrome in critically ill adults: a randomised, parallel-group, multicentre, single-blind controlled trial. Lancet Respir Med. 2015;3:943–52.

8. Cooney RN, Frankenfield DC. Determining energy needs in critically ill patients: equations or indirect calorimeters. Curr Opin Crit Care. 2012;18:174–7.

9. De Waele E, Opsomer T, Honore PM, Diltoer M, Mattens S, Huyghens L, et al. Measured versus calculated resting energy expenditure in critically ill adult patients. Do mathematics match the gold standard? Minerva Anestesiol. 2015;81:272–82.

10. Hoffer LJ, Bistrian BR. Why critically ill patients are protein deprived. JPEN J Parenter Enteral Nutr. 2013;37:300–9.

11. Calder PC. Omega-3 polyunsaturated fatty acids and inflammatory processes: nutrition or pharmacology? Br J Clin Pharmacol. 2013;75:645–62.

12. Singer P, Berger MM, Van den Berghe G, Biolo G, Calder P, Forbes A, et al. ESPEN guidelines on parenteral nutrition: intensive care. Clin Nutr. 2009;28:387–400.

13. Manzanares W, Dhaliwal R, Jiang X, Murch L, Heyland DK. Antioxidant micronutrients in the critically ill: a systematic review and meta-analysis. Crit Care. 2012;16:R66.

14. Manzanares W, Lemieux M, Elke G, Langlois PL, Bloos F, Heyland DK. High-dose intravenous selenium does not improve clinical outcomes in the critically ill: a systematic review and meta-analysis. Crit Care. 2016;20:356.

15. Elke G, van Zanten AR, Lemieux M, McCall M, Jeejeebhoy KN, Kott M, et al. Enteral versus parenteral nutrition in critically ill patients: an updated systematic review and meta-analysis of randomized controlled trials. Crit Care. 2016;20:117.

16. Reintam Blaser A, Starkopf J, Alhazzani W, Berger MM, Casaer MP, Deane AM, et al. Early enteral nutrition in critically ill patients: ESICM clinical practice guidelines. Intensive Care Med. 2017;43:380–98.

17. Doig GS, Simpson F, Sweetman EA, Finfer SR, Cooper DJ, Heighes PT, et al. Early parenteral nutrition in critically ill patients with short-term relative contraindications to early

enteral nutrition: a randomized controlled trial. JAMA. 2013;309:2130–8.

18. Harvey S, Parrott F, Harrison D, et al. Trial of the route of early nutritional support in critically ill adults - Calories Trial. New Engl J Med 2014;371:1673–84.

19. Reignier J, Boisrame-Helms J, Brisard L, et al. Enteral versus parenteral early nutrition in ventilated adults with shock: a randomised, controlled, multicentre, open-label, parallel-group study (NUTRIREA-2). Lancet. 2017. e-pub Nov 8, doi:10.1016/S0140-6736(17)32146-3.

20. Alberda C, Gramlich L, Jones N, Jeejeebhoy K, Day AG, Dhaliwal R, et al. The relationship between nutritional intake and clinical outcomes in critically ill patients: results of an international multicenter observational study. Intensive Care Med. 2009;35:1728–37.

21. Pradelli L, Graf S, Pichard C, Berger MM. Cost-effectiveness of the supplemental parenteral nutrition intervention in intensive care patients. Clin Nutr. 2017.; epub Jan 25, doi:10.1016/j.clnu.2017.01.009

Chapter 2
Nutrition During Prolonged Hemodynamic Instability

Itai Bendavid and Pierre Singer

2.1 Introduction

Periods of starvation and underfeeding are very common in the setting of prolonged critical illness and shock, which constitute catabolic states, mitigated by the sympathetic nervous system, inflammatory mediators, and gut hormones. Practically all patients in states of prolonged shock are underfed, and most are sedated and mechanically ventilated. Energy and protein intake are generally low. The resulting changes in body composition differ across the course of critical illness. We aim to review current knowledge on metabolic changes during prolonged shock and address nutrition treatment issues in this patient population. It must be stressed that most physiologic studies were derived from animal models and caution must be exercised in the interpretation of these data. Patients undergoing extracorporeal membrane oxygenation therapy (ECMO) are discussed in Chap. 3.

I. Bendavid • P. Singer (✉)
Department of General Intensive Care and Institute for Nutrition Research, Rabin Medical Center, Beilinson Hospital, Petah Tikva, Israel

Sackler School of Medicine, Tel Aviv University, Tel Aviv, Israel
e-mail: Psinger@clalit.org.il

© Springer International Publishing AG 2018   15
M.M. Berger (ed.), *Critical Care Nutrition Therapy for Non-nutritionists*, https://doi.org/10.1007/978-3-319-58652-6_2

2.2   Prolonged Hemodynamic Instability

In shock, tissues suffer from a nutrient supply inferior to the tissues' demands. Cardiac function, macro- and microvascular changes, and altered cellular uptake and metabolism play parts in the development of end-organ damage. The prolonged state of hypoperfusion and tissue ischemia leads to multi-organ failure with very high mortality rates. Different types of shock involve different pathophysiological processes. During cardiogenic shock with pump failure, cardiac output is reduced, while systemic resistance varies widely. During septic shock, cardiac output is elevated, but there is actually evidence of reduced stroke volume. The classic "ebb" and "flow" response to shock was described by Cuthberson in 1942 [1]. It classically represented a short-lived period (2–5 days with large variability) characterized by low cardiac output and oxygen consumption followed by a period of hypermetabolism with hyperdynamic circulation.

2.3   Metabolic Changes During Prolonged Shock

Even within a specific type of shock, it is hard to generalize the metabolic adaptations.

The "ebb" phase mentioned above represents an immediate short-lived hypometabolic phase, perhaps designated to conserve energy during insult. It is followed by a more prolonged hypermetabolic phase that may continue for weeks [2]. It must be stressed that different patients may react differently: while in some, an immediate hypercatabolic reaction develops, others show such signs only much later in the course of shock [3]. During this hypercatabolic state, metabolic dysregulation leads to increases in glycolysis, glycemic levels, Krebs cycle activity, fatty acid metabolism, amino acid metabolism, and nitrogen metabolism (urate and polyamines). Another effect is impaired redox homeostasis.

In healthy subjects, the utilization of substrates is largely dictated by nutrient intake from diet as well as time elapsed from the last meal. However, during critical illness, the body turns more to endogenous sources of energy under the effect of stress mechanisms (inflammatory mediators, hormones, sympathetic drive). These act on various sites, including gut function and intracellular metabolic mechanisms. In the early phases of critical illness and shock, this means oxidation of carbohydrates with low metabolism of lipids and protein. However, as the state of critical illness prolongs, glucose utilization drops while lipid oxidation and lean body protein breakdown rise in effect. During prolonged starvation in prolonged critical illness, the resting metabolic rate and tissue catabolism rise, while ketogenesis may in fact remain suppressed [4].

2.4   Carbohydrates and Insulin

Glucose is the main substrate for energy, i.e., ATP production. Glucose uptake, as well as lactate and pyruvate production and uptake, differs widely across patient populations. There is also great variability in the metabolism of carbohydrates in different organ systems; for example, a study [5] looking into ischemic cardiac shock revealed wide variations (both increments and falls) in the levels of lactate and pyruvate. During septic shock, it appears that lactate uptake by the myocardium is increased [6]. In general, many tissues exhibit increased glucose uptake during sepsis when compared to non-septic states with the same insulin levels [7]. Hyperglycemia is a common presentation very early in the course of any type of shock. The mechanisms include the activity of adipose tissue hormones (adiponectin, leptin, resistin), ghrelin released from the gut, and the sympathetic nervous system. Severe hyperglycemia (over 200 mg/dL) and hypoglycemia (even mild, less than 70 mg/dL) have been shown to correlate with increased mortality in various types of shock. This effect is more marked in patients without a medical history of

diabetes mellitus, which is not the case for milder hyperglycemia (141–199 mg/dL) which is considered by most as a proper
reaction to stress. The effects of catecholamines, cytokines,
and counter-regulatory hormones lead to increased hepatic
glucose production and peripheral insulin resistance. Aside
from hyper- and hypoglycemia, increased glucose variability,
the standard deviation of each patient's mean glucose level,
has been strongly correlated with mortality in critically ill
patients. As the state of shock protracts and exacerbates, liver
cells may lose their ability to cope with the metabolic load,
hepatocyte mitochondrial function diminishes, and hyperlactatemia may ensue, a dreaded potentially ominous sign in this
context.

The effects of vasopressors on glucose metabolism have
been studied. Circulating endogenous norepinephrine plays
a part in the metabolic response to stress, including glycemic
levels. However, the effect of exogenous norepinephrine is
very mild and transient [8]. The effect of epinephrine is different as it leads to increased hepatic glucose output and sustained inhibition of glucose uptake. This may in turn lead to
the hyperlactatemia associated with epinephrine as pyruvate
accumulates and reactions shift toward lactate production
instead of pyruvate dehydrogenase complex. None of these
effects are mediated by glucagon. Low-dose vasopressin
does not seem to have any effect on glucose levels or insulin
resistance [9].

2.5   Lipids

Lipids' roles in the body are beyond the scope of this chapter. Compared to carbohydrates, lipids are a less immediate
source of energy, requiring functioning mitochondria and
large amounts of oxygen. Hence, during the initial phases
of critical illness, lipids do not play a major part in energy
production. Triglycerides are hydrolyzed into free fatty acids
and glycerol, regardless of exogenous administration; thus,
fatty acid levels are high during the first days of acute severe
illness. These lipid breakdown products have been implicated

as contributors to end-organ damage. Later in the course of critical illness, fatty acids are converted into ketone bodies in the liver, while fatty acid metabolism in peripheral tissues is increased as well, making lipids more central in energy production in the later phases of critical illness. As prolonged starvation leads to reduced ketogenesis [4], the timing of initiation and composition of exogenous nutrition may have effects on the degrees of lipolysis as well as proteolysis.

The effect of polyunsaturated fatty acids (PUFAs) and their effect on the immune response have been extensively studied. Variations in content of omega-3 and omega-6 (n-3 and n-6, respectively) translate into the formation of different leukotrienes, prostaglandins, and thromboxanes as well as other products with effect on inflammation and its resolution, cell adhesion, and platelet aggregation. The use of "immunonutrition," most commonly a combination of n-3 PUFAs, arginine, and glutamine, has led to conflicting results, with n-3 supplementation found to be harmful on certain studies.

The actions of prolonged infusions of epinephrine and norepinephrine are probably mediated at least partly by the liver. They include increased lipolysis and elevated levels of free fatty acids. Vasopressin's physiologic effects on lipids are in fact opposite, as it regulates various hormones, e.g., insulin and glucagon, and inhibits peripheral tissue lipase, leading to reduced lipolysis and lower plasma levels of free fatty acids.

2.6   Protein

As mentioned, during early phases of critical illness, proteins are not key precursors for energy production in the early phase of critical illness. However, as the state of shock protracts, by mediation of prostaglandins and the ubiquitin-proteasome among others, there is increased proteolysis and gluconeogenesis with rapid and significant loss of lean muscle tissue. During this hypercatabolic state, which may last for a very long period, nutritional support is a double-edged sword as overfeeding may in fact be more harmful than underfeeding. Not only will overfeeding not achieve an increase in muscle mass, but it may also deteriorate muscle function by means such as muscle tissue fatty infiltration, eventually translating into poorer long-term outcome measures. Current good practice emphasizes protein as a major constituent in the nutritional support of the critically ill, comprising about 20% of daily intake and attempting to reach 1.2–2.0 g/kg/day in most patients with the objective to reduce the total negative nitrogen balance and lean muscle tissue loss.

While total protein targets have been better defined, much less is known concerning recommended amino acid composition. As mentioned earlier, glutamine and arginine may exert beneficial anti-inflammatory effects, mainly in postsurgical patients. This effect may be related to glutamine's protective effect on gut mucosa from ischemia-reperfusion injury [10]. However, the administration of glutamine has also been shown to increase succinate levels in the plasma and lungs, potentially exacerbating lung injury with long-term use [11]. In addition, the REDOXS study [12] showed that in most hemodynamically unstable patients, the administration of supra-nutritional doses of glutamine independent of nutrition was associated with increased mortality. This was even more pronounced in presence of kidney or liver failure. Arginine was found to be deficient in prolonged critical illness [13]. Its supplementation may exert beneficial effects such as reduced inflammation and improved nitric oxide production, potentially improving tissue blood supply without affecting hemodynamics [14]. However, arginine is still not recommended for most critically ill patients by the American and European guidelines [15, 16].

2.7   Nutrition and Elevated Lactate Levels

Lactate was traditionally seen as a marker of anaerobic metabolism, mainly due to inadequate oxygen supply. However, in the last decade hyperlactatemia during states of shock has become considered as a marker of aerobic glycolysis [17]. Muscle lactate is actually produced under the effect of epinephrine, released in the bloodstream and used by the liver to produce glucose through gluconeogenesis. The concept of "bad" lactate as a metabolic waste product has evolved to lactate seen as an energy shuttle or "good lactate." It should be used as a marker of adaptive response to shock. Administering lactate in severe head trauma was associated with less episodes of elevated intracranial pressure [18], while in acute heart failure, lactate administration improved cardiac performance [19]. A study on hemodynamically unstable patients with multiple organ failure undergoing continuous renal replacement therapy with lactate used as a buffer demonstrated that lactate is rapidly metabolized, cleared from the blood, and transformed into glucose or oxidized without creating any undesirable effects [20]. Hyperlactatemia by itself should not automatically lead to withholding nutrition but rather to guide resuscitation and introduce nutrition accordingly.

2.8   Nutritional Support During Prolonged Critical Illness and Shock

Feeding the critically ill patient is not a straightforward matter. Many concerns exist regarding timing, route, amount, and composition. Current guidelines advise initiation of enteral nutrition (EN) during the first days as long as hemodynamic stabilization has been achieved, even if requiring vasopressor support. As 25% of patients were still unfed after 4 days, it should be emphasized that the vast majority of shocked patients should still receive nutrition once deterioration had been stopped. The recent ESICM recommendations [21] "suggest using early EN in adult patients with shock receiving vasopressors or inotropes when shock is controlled with fluids and named medications (conditional recommendation based on expert opinion = Grade 2D)." There are no randomized controlled studies, but there was a large observational study [22] including patients receiving early (within 48 h) versus late enteral nutrition after stabilization of shock

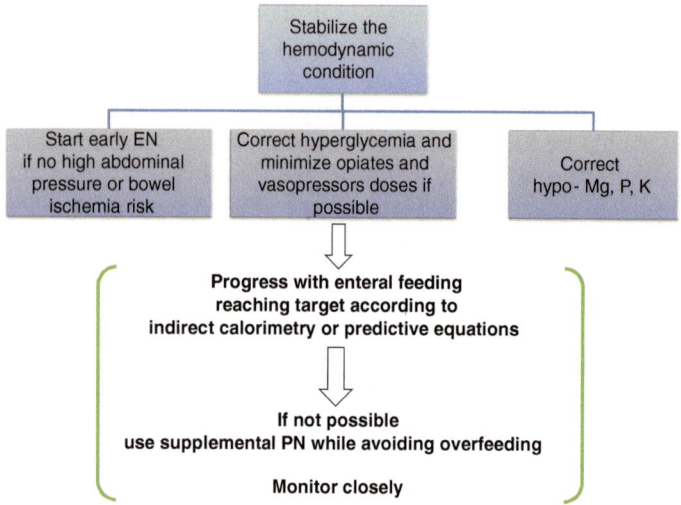

FIGURE 2.1 Flowchart for nutritional therapy in the hemodynamically compromised patient

with fluids and at least one vasopressor, showing an amelioration in survival. The guidelines recommended also "EN should not be started where there is uncontrolled shock and haemodynamic and tissue perfusion goals are not reached (Fig. 2.1)."

The oral route is generally preferred but unfeasible in most if not all patients with prolonged hemodynamic compromise. In general, enteral feeding via a gastric tube is recommended. However, in shocked patients, concerns have been raised following multiple reports of bowel ischemia following enteral feeding, mainly in patients after abdominal surgery for traumatic and non-traumatic pathologies. This is not to say that EN is not advised in shocked patients; in fact, when compared to fasting patients, patients receiving oral or EN showed increased blood flow in the superior mesenteric artery, while patients receiving parenteral nutrition (PN) had reduced splanchnic blood flow [23]. Current evidence shows that gastrointestinal mucosal damage in shock is likely related to tissue hypoxia due to ischemia, the action of inflammatory mediators and reactive oxygen species and deficient nutritional substrates. In the longer term, the avoidance of enteral feeding may actually expose the patient to gut mucosa atrophy and dysfunction, at least partially due to the lack of production of short-chain fatty acids by gut microbiota, leading to bowel mucosa thinning and dysfunction. Hence, as long as there is no specific contraindication, EN should be started early. Still, care must be given to the development of bowel ischemia: its manifestations in patients with a protracted course of shock and critical illness are hard to diagnose as they resemble bacterial sepsis while gastrointestinal symptoms appear late if at all [24, 25]. Patients with advanced atherosclerosis receiving high doses of vasopressors and those undergoing abdominal arterial manipulations as intra-arterial balloon pump or ECMO are at a higher risk. Of note, prospective data concerning feeding in patients on continuous vasopressor therapy is lacking. However, a single prospective observational study showed its feasibility as most could be safely fed and none developed bowel ischemia [26]. In a larger prospective descriptive study on 70 hemodynamically unstable patients after cardiopulmonary bypass revealed no abdominal complications related to EN [27]. Artinian et al. [28] showed, in a retrospective study including 4049 patients, a lower mortality in very sick patients receiving early enteral feeding despite an increase in VAP. The effects of vasopressors and inotropes must be considered: epinephrine has been shown to decrease splanchnic blood flow, while a combination of norepinephrine and dobutamine did not; however, in hypovolemic patients not adequately resuscitated, norepinephrine reduced splanchnic blood flow in a dose-related manner [29]. As current ICU common practice shifts toward a more fluid-restrictive manner of resuscitation, the risk of further reducing blood flow must be considered.

The preferred route for administering EN in most ICU patients is a gastric feeding tube. An enteral (post-pyloric) feeding tube is more expensive and requires more expertise with higher insertion failure rates although its use has led to lower pneumonia rates. Indications for its use are fewer as conditions such as pancreatitis are no longer considered a contraindication to prepyloric feeding. Failure to provide adequate EN is common. The main reasons are high gastric residual volume (GRV), surgical reasons, and patient transport (mainly to the operating theater). However, repeated GRV measurements are no longer recommended as routine, and when used, a patient should be kept fed as long as the GRV is lower than 500 mL.

There is a potential role for markers of bowel function such as citrulline or urine intestinal fatty-acid-binding protein, but their role in guiding therapy according to gut functional integrity remains uncertain. Progression of enteral feeding will be performed according to the ESCIM recommendations [21]. PN should be prescribed when EN cannot be delivered within 4 days [30], although many initiate PN earlier once hemodynamic stability has been achieved. In any case, if the patient was starved for a week or more, special care must be taken to reduce the risk for the development of the refeeding syndrome, i.e., slowly increasing the dose while tightly monitoring electrolyte levels. Specifically for septic shock patients, recent Surviving Sepsis guidelines [31] recommend the initiation of enteral nutrition early and are cautious regarding parenteral nutrition, recommending its initiation only after 7 days if the patient cannot tolerate enteral nutrition. The ESICM recommendations [21] propose to start PN earlier.

As patients in states of prolonged shock and catabolism may have a very large variability in energy demands, it is advisable to guide caloric prescription according to measurement by means of indirect calorimetry. Care should be given to prescribe vitamins and trace elements, and in some patient populations in whom loss is expected to be higher such as burn patients and those undergoing continuous renal replacement therapy, doses may be increased. The surviving sepsis [31] study group did not find any evidence suggesting an advantage for the administration of n-3 fatty acids, glutamine, arginine, carnitine, or high doses of selenium. Recently, a study associating high doses of vitamin C, thiamine, and hydrocortisone has suggested an improvement in survival

[32]. Glucose levels should be monitored closely for the development of hypo- and hyperglycemic states. In most critically ill patients, the range of 140–180 mg/dL (7–10 mmol/L) is considered optimal as lower glycemic targets led to more frequent events of hypoglycemia.

2.9   Conclusions

The critically ill hemodynamically unstable patient is a challenge for nutrition therapy. After intensive resuscitation and stabilization, we recommend to start early enteral feeding cautiously taking into account the risks of ischemic bowel and intraabdominal pressure, as well as gastrointestinal tolerance. This strategy seems associated with clinical advantages. Progression to calorie target ideally defined by indirect calorimetry will be performed according to the patient tolerance to this process. If not achievable enterally, supplemental parenteral nutrition is feasible mainly if not inducing overnutrition. Close monitoring is the key of this treatment, while correction of hyperglycemia, hyperlipidemia, hypokalemia, magnesemia, and phosphatemia is mandatory. Best understanding of the physiology compromise of these patients is the key for successful nutritional therapy.

References

1. Cuthbertson D. Post-shock metabolic response. Lancet. 1942;239:433–7.
2. Jeschke MG, Gaguglitz GG, Kulp GA, et al. Long-term persistence of the pathophysiologic response to severe stress. PLoS One. 2011;6(7):e21245.
3. D'Alessandro A, Moore HB, Moore EE, et al. Early hemorrhage triggers metabolic responses that build up during prolonged shock. Am J Physiol Regul Integr Comp Physiol. 2015;308(12):R1034–44.
4. Chioléro R, Revelly JP, Tappy L. Energy metabolism in sepsis and injury. Nutrition. 1997;13(9 Suppl):45S–51S.

5. Mueller H, Ayres SM, Gregory JJ, et al. Hemodynamics, coronary blood flow and myocardial metabolism in coronary shock; response of 1-norepinephrine and isoproterenol. J Clin Invest. 1970;49(10):1885–902.

6. Dhainaut JF, Huyghebaert MF, Mondallier JF, et al. Coronary hemodynamics and myocardial metabolism of lactate, free fatty acids, glucose, and ketones in patients with septic shock. Circulation. 1987;75(3):533–41.

7. Lang CH, Dobrescu C, Mészáros K. Insulin-mediated glucose uptake by individual tissues during sepsis. Metabolism. 1990;39(10):1096–107.

8. Saccà L, Morrone G, Cicala M, et al. Influence of epinephrine, norepinephrine and isoproterenol on glucose homeostasis in normal man. J Clin Endocrinol Metab. 1980;50(4):680–4.

9. Tsuneyoshi I, Yamada H, Kakihana Y, et al. Hemodynamic and metabolic effects of low-dose vasopressin infusions in vasodilatory septic shock. Crit Care Med. 2001;29(3):487–93.

10. Kozar RA, Schultz SG, Bick RJ, et al. Enteral glutamine but not alanine maintains small bowel barriers function after ischemia/reperfusion injury in rats. Shock. 2004;21(5):433–7.

11. Slaughter AL, D'Alessandro A, Moore EE, et al. Glutamine metabolism drives succinate accumulation in plasma and the lung during hemorrhagic shock. J Trauma Acute Care Surg. 2016;81(6):1012–9.

12. Heyland D, Muscedere J, Wischmeyer PE, et al. A randomized controlled trial of glutamine and antioxidants in critically ill patients. N Engl J Med. 2016;368(16):1489–97.

13. Luiking YC, Poeze M, Ramsay G, et al. Reduced citrulline production in sepsis is related to diminished de novo arginine and nitric oxide production. Am J Clin Nutr. 2009;89(1):142–52.

14. Luiking YC, Poeze M, Deutz NE. Arginine infusion in patients with septic shock increases nitric oxide production without hemodynamic instability. Clin Sci (Lond). 2015;128(1):57–67.

15. Singer P, Berger MM, Van den Bergh G, et al. ESPEN guidelines on parenteral nutrition: intensive care. Clin Nutr. 2009;28(4):387–400.

16. McClave SA, Taylor BE, Martindale RG, et al. Guidelines for the provision and assessment of nutrition support therapy in the adult critically ill patient: Society of Critical Care Medicine (SCCM) and American Society for Parenteral and Enteral Nutrition (A.S.P.E.N.). JPEN J Parenter Enteral Nutr. 2016;40(2): 159–211.

17. Levy B. Lactate and shock state: the metabolic view. Curr Opin Crit Care. 2006;12:315–21.
18. Ichai C, Payen JF, Orban JC, et al. Half-molar sodium lactate infusion to prevent intracranial hypertensive episodes in severe traumatic brain injured patients: a randomized controlled trial. Intensive Care Med. 2013;39(8):1413–22.
19. Nalos M, Leverve X, Huang S, et al. Half-molar sodium lactate infusion improves cardiac performance in acute heart failure: a pilot randomised controlled clinical trial. Crit Care. 2014;18(2):R4.
20. Bollman MD, Revelly JP, Tappy L, et al. Effect of bicarbonate and lactate buffer on glucose and lactate metabolism during hemodiafiltration in patients with multiple organ failure. Intensive Care Med. 2004;30:1103–10.
21. Reinthan Blaser A, Starkopf J, Alhazzani W, et al. Early enteral nutrition in critically ill patients: ESICM clinical practice guidelines. Intensive Care Med. 2017;43(3):380–98.
22. Reignier J, Darmon M, Sonneville R, et al. Impact of early nutrition and feeding route on outcomes of mechanically ventilated patients with shock: a post hoc marginal structural model study. Intensive Care Med. 2015;41(5):875–86.
23. Gatt M, MacFie J, Anderson AD, et al. Changes in superior mesenteric artery blood flow after oral, enteral and parenteral feeding in humans. Crit Care Med. 2009;37(1):171–6.
24. Melis M, Fischera A, Ferguson MK. Bowel necrosis associated with early jejunal tube feeding: a complication of postoperative enteral nutrition. Arch Surg. 2006;141(7):701–4.
25. Marvin R, McKinley BA, McQuiggan M, et al. Nonocclusive bowel necrosis occurring in critically ill trauma patients receiving enteral nutrition manifests no reliable clinical signs for early detection. Am J Surg. 2000;179(1):7–12.
26. Flordelis Lasierra JL, Pérez-Vela JL, Umezawa Makikado LD, et al. Early enteral nutrition in patients with hemodynamic failure following cardiac surgery. JPEN J Parenter Enteral Nutr. 2015;39(2):154–62.
27. Berger MM, Revelly JP, Cayeux MC, et al. Enteral nutrition in critically ill patients with severe hemodynamic failure after cardiopulmonary bypass. Clin Nutr. 2005;24:124–32.
28. Artinian V, Krayem H, DiGiovine B. Effects of early enteral feeding on the outcome of critically ill mechanically ventilated medical patients. Chest. 2006;129:960–7.
29. Allen JM. Vasoactive substances and their effects on nutrition in the critically ill patients. Nutr Clin Pract. 2012;27:335–9.

30. Weimann A, Felbinger TW. Gastrointestinal dysmotility in the critically ill: a role for nutrition. Curr Opin Clin Nutr Metab Care. 2016 (Epub ahead of print).
31. Rhodes A, Evans LE, Alhazzani W, et al. Surviving sepsis campaign: international guidelines for management of sepsis and septic shock: 2016. Intensive Care Med. 2017;43(3):304–77.
32. Marik PE, Khangoora V, Rivera R, Hooper MH, et al. Hydrocortisone, vitamin C, and thiamine for the treatment of severe sepsis and septic shock: a retrospective before-after study. Chest. 2017;151(6):1229–38.

Further Reading

1. Wells DL. Provision of enteral nutrition during vasopressor therapy for hemodynamic instability: an evidence-based review. Nutr Clin Pract. 2012;27(4):521–6.
2. Khalid I, Doshi P, DiGiovine B. Early enteral nutrition and outcomes of critically ill patients treated with vasopressors and mechanical ventilation. Am J Crit Care. 2010;19(3):261–8.
3. Mentec H, Dupont H, Bocchetti M, Cani P, Ponche F, Bleichner G. Upper digestive intolerance during enteral nutrition in critically ill patients: frequency, risk factors, and complications. Crit Care Med. 2001;29(10):1955–61.
4. Fontaine E, Müller MJ. Adaptive alterations in metabolism: practical consequences on energy requirements in the severely ill patient. Curr Opin Clin Nutr Metab Care. 2011;14(2):171–5.
5. Cresci G, Cúe J. The patient with circulatory shock: to feed or not to feed? Nutr Clin Pract. 2008;23(5):501–9.

Chapter 3
ECMO Patients

Tobias Wollersheim, Michael C. Müller, and Steffen Weber-Carstens

3.1 Extracorporeal Membrane Oxygenation: Venovenous ECMO and Venoarterial ECMO

Intensive care teams are running a growing number of Extracorporeal membrane oxygenation (ECMO) therapies for pulmonary and cardiac support every year, reaching a total of almost 8000 therapies in 2015 [1]. Even after clinical establishment and tremendous technological improvements [2], these therapies are restricted to the sickest and most vulnerable patients and often remain a salvage therapy resulting in mortality rates of over 40% [1]. Specific research on ECMO and nutrition is mainly missing, but there is no reason to believe ECMO patients

T. Wollersheim* (✉) • M.C. Müller • S. Weber-Carstens*
Department of Anesthesiology and Operative Intensive Care Medicine, Charité—Universitätsmedizin Berlin, Campus Virchow-Klinikum, Augustenburger Platz 1, Berlin 13353, Germany

*Berlin Institute of Health (BIH),
Anna-Louisa-Karsch-Str. 2, Berlin 10178, Germany
e-mail: tobias.wollersheim@charite.de

© Springer International Publishing AG 2018   29
M.M. Berger (ed.), *Critical Care Nutrition Therapy for Non-nutritionists*, https://doi.org/10.1007/978-3-319-58652-6_3

could not profit from optimal nutrition. This chapter will outline the specific issues of ECMO patients, trying to answer the mainly two questions and their clinical consequences:

1. What does the ECMO therapy imply for the nutritional needs?
2. Which particular problems do we need to address when feeding ECMO patients?

3.2   What Does ECMO Therapy Imply for Nutritional Needs?

3.2.1   Does the ECMO Therapy Itself Influence the Energetic Needs?

The influence of the extracorporeal circulation on the energetic needs is largely uninvestigated. A biomaterial-related systemic inflammatory response has been witnessed in relation to ECMO and cardiopulmonary bypass (CBP) treatments [3]. Inflammatory response (represented by Il-6 levels) has been linked to increased resting energy expenditure (REE) in a pediatric study after CPB [4]: however, another study found no influence of infection on REE [5]. In adult ECMO patients, no significant influence has been described for the (venovenous ECMO) vvECMO on REE in a matched group of ARDS patient comparison or using an intraindividual approach (ECMO compared with post ECMO) [6]. Also, a study comparing the REE of eight Venoarterial ECMO (vaECMO) neonates with ten postoperative neonates without ECMO did not find a significant difference, thus not supporting a claimed hypermetabolic state in earlier research in neonatal ECMO [7] (Fig. 3.1).

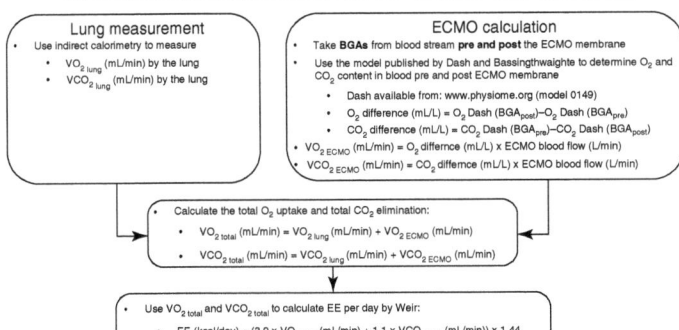

FIGURE 3.1 Flow chart showing the MEEP protocol. O_2 oxygen, CO_2 carbon dioxide, VO_2 oxygen uptake (mL/min), VCO_2 carbon dioxide elimination (mL/min), *BGA* blood gas analyses, *pre ECMO* efferent ECMO bloodstream before the membrane, *post ECMO* afferent ECMO bloodstream after passing the membrane, *EE* energy expenditure, *lung* indicates values of the lung, *ECMO* indicates values from the ECMO, *total* indicates total values after summing up lung and ECMO values. Dash and Bassingthwaighte: the model allows to determine the O_2 and CO_2 content of blood under consideration of pH, pO_2, pCO_2, Hct, SpO_2, temperature, and 2,3-BPG. For standard BGAs we set 2,3-BPG to normal values (4.65 mmol/L). Reprinted from [6] with permission from Elsevier

3.2.2   Does the ECMO Circuit Interact with Macro- and Micronutritional Components?

The influence of the circuit and the membrane itself on different molecules has been researched. Sequestration has been described for various drugs, and a reduction of important trace elements (e.g., selenium, copper, and zinc in CPB) was witnessed [8]. An ex vivo study [9] on ECMO circuits filled with human blood found a significant loss of the essential amino acids leucine and vitamins A and E but encouragingly found most other macro- and micronutrients stable over 24 h. Over all the clinical impact of these findings is yet unclear, especially as inflammation has influence on levels of selenium, copper, and zinc also without ECMO treatment [10] and vice versa ECMO could cause inflammation [3].

3.2.3 Does ECMO per se Influence the Integrity of the Intestine?

Animal studies observed deterioration of the mucosal barrier after a few hours on ECMO. An observation of 16 neonates found increased intestinal permeability via sugar absorption on vaECMO and no significant change after the initiation of enteral nutrition (EN) [11]. A newer study by Ni et al. addressed these findings in a porcine ARDS model and found an initial aggravation of intestinal injury in the ECMO group and a protective effect on the mucosa at the later stage of treatment, as well as a decreased mortality in the treatment group [12]. The implications of these findings for humans and especially adult ECMO patients remain largely uninvestigated.

3.3 Which Particular Problems Do We Need to Address When Feeding ECMO Patients?

3.3.1 How to Approach the Energy Needs of ECMO Patients: Equations vs. Measuring

Of over 200 published predictive equations, no single one could be suggested in the guidelines published by the ASPEN as being more accurate than the others in ICU patients, especially in underweight or obese patients [13]. De Waele et al. compared equations to indirect calorimetry in 259 critically ill, ventilated patients and found all equations insufficiently accurate, with only Swinamer and Penn State 2010 reaching a correlation coefficient (R^2) > 0.5 [14]. Measuring the REE in 20 patients undergoing ECMO with a new approach showed a similar inaccuracy of all published equations [6]. The ASPEN guidelines suggest choosing a published predictive equation or 25–30 kcal/kg/day for critically ill adult patients, and the ESPEN guidelines (2009) recommend 20–25 kcal/kg/day in critically ill adult patients [15]. Scientific research focusing on the critically ill group of adult patients on ECMO is largely missing, implying that these suggestions seem to be the best treatment option for the ECMO patients. For the special group of neonatal ECMO, the 2010 ASPEN guideline for neonates [16] recommends early EN (EEN) or PN aiming for 100–120 kcal/kg/day. As a consequence of the well-researched inaccuracy of all formulas, guidelines and studies suggest an objective approach of the caloric needs via indirect calorimetry [13–15]. Classic indirect calorimetry as the gold standard for determining REE is not possible for patients on ECMO because of the missing possibility to measure the gas exchange over the membrane. Several promising approaches to overcome these technical difficulties were carried out: measurement of CO_2 production via C^{13} isotopic measurements [7], mass spectrometry of the respiratory and efflux gas [17], and simultaneous indirect calorimetry from the ECMO and the lung [18]. We described a novel and technically simple method [6] using standard indirect calorimetry and blood samples from before and after the membrane oxygenator. The results of the blood gas analysis from the blood samples are expressed as absolute O_2 and CO_2 volumes per liter blood, very exactly calculated via a spreadsheet adopting a method by Dash and Bassingthwaighte [19]. In a next step, the gas volume difference between before and after the ECMO membrane is calculated and multiplicated with the ECMO flow per minute, expressing the metabolic work of the ECMO as O_2 mL/min and CO_2 mL/min. The metabolism of the body now can be expressed by first summing up O_2 and CO_2 values from ECMO and indirect calorimetry and then inserting the results into the standard EE formula by Weir [20].

Outstanding from all methods published before is the lacking need for any technical equipment besides an indirect calorimetry and a blood gas analysis machine, which is omnipresent in ICUs, or potentially dangerous modifications to the ECMO filter.

The data of the pilot trial was published in 2017 with 20 patients, while all published data [7, 17, 18, 21, 22] in the three decades before presented 21 patients in total. We concluded that the translation of this approach into clinical routine is easy, making the measuring the energetic needs also possible for patients on ECMO. Furthermore, chances are that measurement of DO_2 and VCO_2 during ECMO could be also a powerful research tool, potentially revealing undiscovered pathophysiological links, maybe also leading to optimized therapy in the future.

3.3.2   Which Feeding Route Is the Best? When to Attempt Post-Pyloric Feeding?

Enteral nutrition for ECMO patients through the commonly used gastric tube has been described in several studies as safe and feasible [23], even when starting early (average 13 h after ICU admission [24]). Commonly described problems include the frequent interruption of EN for diagnostic or therapeutic procedures and high gastric residual volumes (GRV) resulting in calorie deficits [23]. While prokinetics were commonly used, postpyloric feeding was only reported as necessary on 10% of the study days [23].

No data on the widely discussed topic EN vs. PN exists for ECMO patients. Following recommendations for general ICU collectives aiming for EEN is recommended, and in case of contraindications, the use of PN is suggested [13, 25].

3.3.3   ECMO and Lipids: What to Consider?

Unlike the normal patient, ECMO patients have an artificial capillary system which needs to be taken into consideration. Administering fat emulsions while on ECMO, for nutritional needs but also as lipid rescue for poisoning, has been associated with increased clotting, layering, and agglutination in the circuit, also despite sufficient anticoagulation [26]. Also the route of administration seems to be important: an increased probability of layering was observed when given fatty infusions directly into the circuit [26]. Even though only limited research on this topic is published, administering fatty infusions directly in the ECMO circuit should be avoided when possible, and the circuit should be closely checked for layering or clots independent from the administration route.

3.3.4   When Is the Best Time to Initiate Feeding?

According to the recent guidelines by ESICM [25] and recommendations for general ICU patients, early enteral nutrition within 24–48 h is suggested for the ECMO patients (in absence of uncontrolled shock, hypoxemia or acidosis, abdominal compartment or bowel obstruction/ischemia, etc.). For non-ECMO sepsis patients, the full caloric target can be advanced after successful initiation of EEN or trophic feeding to the full target energy, as tolerated after 24–48 h.

3.3.5   What Kind of Nutrition Is Most Appropriate?

A standard high-protein formula providing 1.2–2.0 g/kg/day is most appropriate, assuring that the protein target is reached; if needed, this can be prepared in a volume-restricted preparation (1.5–2 kcal/mL) to prevent volume overload [13]. Furthermore, the preparation should of course meet the micro- and macronutrient content described in Sect. 3.1.

3.3.6   Can We Feed During Prone Positioning and While Neuromuscular Blockade?

Encouraging studies suggest the use of prone positioning in ARDS patients, sometimes also in combination with ECMO. Studies suggest feeding is safe during prone position

[27], and the ESICM guidelines for non-ECMO patients suggest not to delay EN because of prone positioning [25]; yet prokinetics and postpyloric feeding should be considered early. ECMO patients are sometimes treated with neuromuscular blockers. Tamion et al. did not find significant influence on gastric emptying [28], and guidelines for non-ECMO patients do not suggest delaying nutrition. Nevertheless, necessary deep sedation increases the rate of EN intolerance [25], while the administration of neuromuscular blockers per se in the treatment of ARDS patients is controversial and beyond the scope of this chapter.

3.4   Conclusion

Patients undergoing ECMO therapy are usually among the most severely ill patients, and their nutrition needs special attention. The difficult task of defining a caloric target remains, despite its extreme importance,- and we strongly suggest the use of measurement techniques. Furthermore, there is no main difference in therapy and administration compared to other ICU patients as recommended in the recent nutrition guidelines.

Beyond the nutrition itself, it should be taken into consideration that the combination of optimal nutrition and exercise in critical illness has been hypothesized to have the greatest impact on the physical recovery [29].

References

1. Thiagarajan RR, Barbaro RP, Rycus PT, Mcmullan DM, Conrad SA, Fortenberry JD, et al. Extracorporeal life support organization registry international report 2016. ASAIO. 2017;63(1):60–7.
2. Ramakrishna H. Extracorporeal circulation-from cardiopulmonary bypass to extracorporeal membrane oxygenation and mechanical cardiac assist device therapy: a constant evolution. Ann Card Anaesth. 2015;18(2):133–7.
3. Millar JE, Fanning JP, McDonald CI, McAuley DF, Fraser JF. The inflammatory response to extracorporeal membrane

oxygenation (ECMO): a review of the pathophysiology. Crit Care. 2016;20(1):387.

4. Floh AA, Nakada M, La Rotta G, Mah K, Herridge JE, Van Arsdell G, et al. Systemic inflammation increases energy expenditure following pediatric cardiopulmonary bypass. Pediatr Crit Care Med. 2015;16(4):343–51.

5. Raurich JM, Ibáñez J, Marsé P, Riera M, Homar X. Resting energy expenditure during mechanical ventilation and its relationship with the type of lesion. J Parenter Enteral Nutr. 2007;31(1):58–62.

6. Wollersheim T, Frank S, Müller MC, Skrypnikov V, Carbon NM, Pickerodt PA, et al. Measuring Energy Expenditure in extracorporeal lung support Patients (MEEP) — Protocol, feasibility and pilot trial - Clinical Nutrition. Available online 16 January 2017, ISSN 0261–5614, https://doi.org/10.1016/j.clnu.2017.01.001.

7. Keshen TH, Miller RG, Jahoor F, Jaksic T. Stable isotopic quantitation of protein metabolism and energy expenditure in neonates on-and post-extracorporeal life support. J Pediatr Surg. 1997;32(7):958–63.

8. Mcdonald CI, Fung YL, Shekar K, Diab SD, Dunster KR, Passmore MR, et al. The impact of acute lung injury, ECMO and transfusion on oxidative stress and plasma selenium levels in an ovine model. J Trace Elem Med Biol. 2015;30:4–10.

9. Estensen K, Shekar K, Robins E, McDonald C, Barnett AG, Fraser JF. Macro- and micronutrient disposition in an ex vivo model of extracorporeal membrane oxygenation. Intensive Care Med Exp. 2014;2(1):29.

10. Ghashut RA, McMillan DC, Kinsella J, Vasilaki AT, Talwar D, Duncan A. The effect of the systemic inflammatory response on plasma zinc and selenium adjusted for albumin. Clin Nutr. 2016;35(2):381–7.

11. Piena M, Albers MJ, Van Haard PM, Gischler S, Tibboel D. Introduction of enteral feeding in neonates on extracorporeal membrane oxygenation after evaluation of intestinal permeability changes. J Pediatr Surg. 1998;33(1):30–4.

12. Ni L, Chen Q, Zhu K, Shi J, Shen J, Gong J, et al. The influence of extracorporeal membrane oxygenation therapy on intestinal mucosal barrier in a porcine model for post-traumatic acute respiratory distress syndrome. J Cardiothorac Surg. 2015;10:20.

13. McClave SA, Taylor BE, Martindale RG, Warren MM, Johnson DR, Braunschweig C, et al. Guidelines for the provision and assessment of nutrition support therapy in the adult criti-

cally ill patient: Society of Critical Care Medicine (SCCM) and American Society for Parenteral and Enteral Nutrition (A.S.P.E.N.). J Parenter Enteral Nutr. 2016;40(2):159–211.

14. De Waele E, Opsomer T, Honoré PM, Diltoer M, Mattens S, Huyghens L, et al. Measured versus calculated resting energy expenditure in critically ill adult patients. Do mathematics match the gold standard? Minerva Anestesiol. 2015;81(3):272–82.

15. Singer P, Berger MM, Van den Berghe G, Biolo G, Calder P, Forbes A, et al. ESPEN guidelines on parenteral nutrition: intensive care. Clin Nutr. 2009;28(4):387–400.

16. Jaksic T, Hull MA, Modi BP, Ching YA, George D, Compher C, et al. A.S.P.E.N. Clinical guidelines: nutrition support of neonates supported with extracorporeal membrane oxygenation. JPEN J Parenter Enteral Nutr. 2010;34(3):247–53.

17. Cheypesh A, Yu X, Li J. Measurement of systemic oxygen consumption in patients during extracorporeal membrane oxygenation—description of a new method and the first clinical observations. Perfusion. 2014;29(1):57–62.

18. De Waele E, van Zwam K, Mattens S, Staessens K, Diltoer M, Honoré PM, et al. Measuring resting energy expenditure during extracorporeal membrane oxygenation: preliminary clinical experience with a proposed theoretical model. Acta Anaesthesiol Scand. 2015;59(10):1296–302.

19. Dash RK, Bassingthwaighte JB. Erratum to: blood HbO_2 and $HbCO_2$ dissociation curves at varied O_2, CO_2, pH, 2,3-DPG and temperature levels. Ann Biomed Eng. 2010;38(4):1683–701.

20. Weir JB. New methods for calculating metabolic rate with special reference to protein metabolism. J Physiol. 1949;109(1–2): 1–9.

21. Cilley RE, Wesley JR, Zwischenberger JB, Bartlett RH. Gas exchange measurements in neonates treated with extracorporeal membrane oxygenation. J Pediatr Surg. 1988;23(4):306–11.

22. Li X, Yu X, Cheypesh A, Li J. Non-invasive measurements of energy expenditure and respiratory quotient by respiratory mass spectrometry in children on extracorporeal membrane oxygenation—a pilot study: thoughts and progress. Artif Organs. 2015;39(9):815–9.

23. Ridley EJ, Davies AR, Robins EJ, Lukas G, Bailey MJ, Fraser JF, et al. Nutrition therapy in adult patients receiving extracorporeal membrane oxygenation: a prospective, multicentre, observational study. Crit Care Resusc J Australas Acad Crit Care Med. 2015;17(3):183–9.

24. Ferrie S, Herkes R, Forrest P. Nutrition support during extracorporeal membrane oxygenation (ECMO) in adults: a retrospective audit of 86 patients. Intensive Care Med. 2013;39(11):1989–94.

25. Reintam Blaser A, Starkopf J, Alhazzani W, Berger MM, Casaer MP, Deane AM, et al. Early enteral nutrition in critically ill patients: ESICM clinical practice guidelines. Intensive Care Med. 2017;43(3):380–98.

26. Buck ML, Wooldridge P, Ksenich RA. Comparison of methods for intravenous infusion of fat emulsion during extracorporeal membrane oxygenation. Pharmacotherapy. 2005;25(11):1536–40.

27. Linn DD, Beckett RD, Foellinger K. Administration of enteral nutrition to adult patients in the prone position. Intensive Crit Care Nurs. 2015;31(1):38–43.

28. Tamion F, Hamelin K, Duflo A, Girault C, Richard J-C, Bonmarchand G. Gastric emptying in mechanically ventilated critically ill patients: effect of neuromuscular blocking agent. Intensive Care Med. 2003;29(10):1717–22.

29. Heyland DK, Stapleton RD, Mourtzakis M, Hough CL, Morris P, Deutz NE, et al. Combining nutrition and exercise to optimize survival and recovery from critical illness: conceptual and methodological issues. Clin Nutr. 2016;35(5):1196–206.

Chapter 4
Gastro-Intestinal Failure

Annika Reintam-Blaser
and Heleen M. Oudemans-van Straaten

4.1 Introduction

In critically ill patients, gastrointestinal (GI) dysfunction is multifaceted, varying in origin (primary abdominal pathology or consequence of systemic disease) and severity (from self-limiting to life-threatening), affecting different parts of the GI tract and often having complex clinical presentation (motility disorders, discontinuity of the GI tract, infection, etc.). International consensus groups have suggested different approaches defining acute gastrointestinal injury (AGI) with four grades of severity [1] or intestinal failure (IF) in three types depending on duration of parenteral substitution of fluids, electrolytes and nutrients [2, 3].

A. Reintam-Blaser (✉)
Intensive Care, Lucerne Cantonal Hospital, Lucerne, Switzerland
University of Tartu, Tartu, Estonia
e-mail: annika.reintam.blaser@ut.ee

H.M. Oudemans-van Straaten
Department of Intensive Care, VU University Medical Center,
Amsterdam, The Netherlands

© Springer International Publishing AG 2018   41
M.M. Berger (ed.), *Critical Care Nutrition Therapy*
for Non-nutritionists, https://doi.org/10.1007/978-3-319-58652-6_4

The different classifications of acute GI dysfunction are presented in Table 4.1. Notably, GI syndromes are not specific; they may be caused by primary GI pathology or GI dysfunction secondary to systemic disease. Malabsorption or maldigestion, intestinal microbiota dysregulation and gut barrier failure are other manifestations of AGI being part of different syndromes mentioned below. Unfortunately, bedside tools to monitor these conditions are lacking [4]. Because none of the classifications is perfect, we suggest a practical approach assessing clinical symptoms/syndromes and underlying pathophysiological mechanisms as presented below.

We address *acute GI injury (AGI)* and *acute protracted intestinal failure (IF)* separately and specifically describe those clinical scenarios where practitioners often question timing and route of nutritional intervention.

4.2   Acute GI Injury

4.2.1   Specific Characteristics and Nutritional Implications of GI Syndromes

The main characteristics, mechanisms and management of the most common GI symptoms and syndromes are discussed below and in Table 4.2.

4.2.1.1   Gastroparesis

Clinical signs of gastroparesis include anorexia and vomiting, hampering of oral intake and EN. Diagnosis of gastroparesis in the ICU is usually based on large gastric residual volumes (GRV). Alternatively, gastric ultrasound can be used [5]. A randomized study showed that not measuring GRV was not inferior to routine GRV monitoring in terms of development of ventilator-associated pneumonia [6]. However, this study included patients with established enteral nutrition (EN) and excluded GI surgery patients. Even though GRV is neither specific nor sensitive for gastric emptying, removal of gastric

TABLE 4.1 Classifications of acute GI dysfunction

Origin	Time course [2, 3]	Severity [1]
Primary AGI — is associated with primary disease or direct injury to organs of the GI system [1]	Acute (IF type I) — occurs during the acute phase of (critical) illness, often together with other organ dysfunctions.	Risk (AGI Grade I) — GI symptoms after an insult, self-limiting
Secondary AGI — develops as the consequence of a host response in critical illness without primary pathology in the GI system [1]		Dysfunction (AGI Grade II) — requires interventions, several/severe symptoms
Manifestations of primary and secondary AGI may be similar		
GI syndromes *with or without primary abdominal pathology*	Intrinsic GI/abdominal diseases	Lasts for days, may be self-limiting
		Failure (AGI Grade III) — symptoms persist or progress despite interventions, worsening multiple organ failure
Gastroparesis	Bowel obstruction	
Paralytic ileus	Bowel discontinuity	
Bowel oedema	Bowel ischemia	
Bowel distension	Peritonitis/intra-abdominal infection	
Colonic ileus/Ogilvie's syndrome	(Retro)peritoneal hematoma	Failure causing distant organ failure (AGI Grade IV) — dramatically manifested GI failure, immediately life-threatening
	GI bleeding	
Diarrhoea	Acute (entero)colitis	
Intestinal mucosal ischemia	Direct injury to the GI tract (trauma and/or surgery)	
Intra-abdominal hypertension	Transformed continuity of the GI tract (post-surgery)	
	Short bowel syndrome	
	High-output ileostoma	
	(High-output) external intestinal fistula	
	Anastomotic leakage/internal fistula	
	Severe acute pancreatitis	

AGI acute gastrointestinal injury [1], IF intestinal failure [2, 3]

TABLE 4.2 Characteristics, nutritional implications, management and monitoring in different clinical presentations of acute GI dysfunction/failure

Syndrome/mechanism	Symptoms/consequences	Management strategy and nutritional implications	Monitoring
		GI symptoms and syndromes with or without primary abdominal pathology	
Gastroparesis	Vomiting Large gastric residual volumes (GRV) Aspiration	If GRV >500 mL/6 h—no oral or enteral nutrition [7]. Exclude obstruction Start prokinetics: erythromycin 100–250 mg × 2–3 and metoclopramide 10 mg × 3 (1–2 if renal insufficiency). Limit for 3 days. Minimize factors impairing gastric emptying and increasing risk of aspiration (opioids, flat head of bed, etc.). Consider laxatives. If no effect within 24 h, consider jejunal EN. If GRV <500 mL/6 h, start EN[b]. If GRV persistently >200 mL/6 h, consider prokinetics [1]	GRV or repeated gastric ultrasound Clinical assessment[a]
Paralytic ileus Bowel distension/dilatation Ogilvie's syndrome	– No passage [1], abdominal distension, abnormal bowel sounds, elevated intra-abdominal pressure (IAP ≥12 mmHg) – Small bowel diameter >6 cm, caecum >9 cm [1] – No passage, acute severe colonic distension, tenderness over caecum and right colon [10]	If paralytic ileus with or without bowel distension, but GRV <500 mL/6 h and IAP <20 mmHg—start EN 10 mL/h via gastric tube [7]. Correct electrolyte levels. Increase EN cautiously (e.g. by 10 mL/h in 12–24 h). Add prokinetics as above if GRV persistently 200–500 mL/6 h. Add neostigmine i/v infusion 0.4–0.8 mg/h (dose up to 2 mg) if caecum diameter reaches 8–10 cm [11]. Consider endoscopic decompression if not resolved after 48 h. Consider surgery if bowel distension leads to ACS or perforation. Consider supplemental PN after 4–7 days	IAP Organ dysfunctions Lactate levels (risk of ischemia) Bowel diameter if distension clinically not resolved Neostigmine side-effects

Diarrhoea	Liquid stools 3 or more times/day with total stool volume >200 g/day or >250 mL/day [13]. Loss of fluids, electrolytes and nutrients	Stop laxatives. Identify the cause. Exclude/treat *C. difficile* infection: metronidazole and/or vancomycin according to the local protocol [13]. Consider pancreatic exocrine insufficiency and bile acid malabsorption. Check medication list [13]. Start gastric EN 10–20 mL/h, increase cautiously [7]. If diarrhoea clearly worsens with increase of EN, keep hypocaloric EN [12]. Replace fluids, electrolytes and trace elements i/v. Consider PN if malabsorption suspected	Stool frequency, appearance, volume Electrolytes Volume and acid-base status Fat content in stool
Bowel hypoperfusion	Nonspecific, variable abdominal symptoms (e.g. bowel paralysis or diarrhoea), hyperlactatemia Haematoschisis Mucosal ischemic lesions in endoscopy	If no overt transmural ischemia — start EN 10 mL/h and progress very cautiously (e.g. 10 mL/h in 12–24 h) [7]. Risk of ischemia (e.g. abdominal aortic surgery) or mucosal ischemic lesions without peritoneal signs are no contraindications to trophic EN [7]	Clinical assessment[a] Blood lactate levels, serum glucose
Intestinal oedema	Oedema observed in direct observation during surgery or diffuse bowel wall thickening in CT scan after large-volume fluid resuscitation	If severe oedema is accompanied with bowel distension — delay EN for 24 h. Start EN with 10 mL/h and progress cautiously (e.g. 10 mL/h in 12–24 h). Aim negative fluid balance when stable	Clinical assessment[a]

(continued)

TABLE 4.2 (continued)

Syndrome/mechanism	Symptoms/consequences	Management strategy and nutritional implications	Monitoring
Intra-abdominal hypertension	IAP 12 mmHg or higher (measured supine, at end-expirium, with relaxed abdominal muscles) [17]	Start gastric EN 10–20 mL/h if GRV <500 mL and IAP <20 mmHg [7]. Increase 10 mL/h 12-hourly if IAP and GRV are not increasing	GRV IAP
Abdominal compartment syndrome (ACS)	Abdominal distension, IAP >20 mmHg with new/worsening organ dysfunction [17]	Lower IAP: gastric decompression, drain fluid collections/ascites, aim for negative fluid balance, optimize analgesia and sedation [17]. No EN until solved Consider surgical decompression if conservative management not successful and organ failures worsening [17]. Try EN[b] after decompression	IAP Organ dysfunctions Lactate levels (risk of ischemia)
Intrinsic GI/abdominal diseases			
Direct injury to the GI tract Abdominal surgery Abdominal trauma	All previously described symptoms are possible Local bowel oedema is possible	Feeding over surgical jejunostomy after oesophageal surgery. If no jejunostomy performed, start clear fluids orally strictly in sitting position 24 h after surgery. In other cases of GI surgery or trauma, if bowel continuity intact, GRV <500 mL and IAP <20 mmHg, start oral nutrition or gastric EN[b] [7]	GRV Clinical assessment[a] Lactate levels (risk of ischemia)

Bowel obstruction Bowel ischemia Bowel discontinuity	– Abdominal pain, commonly with distension – Abdominal pain with/without distension, hyperlactataemia, hypoglycaemia, diarrhoea, sepsis – No specific symptoms if damage control	Surgical management. No oral or enteral nutrition Early PN (start 25–50% of needs, reach goal by day 4) only if EN not anticipated within 7 days or severe caloric deficit before ICU. Otherwise (supplemental) PN from days 4 to 7	Clinical assessment[a] Blood lactate levels, serum glucose K, Mg, phosphate (cave refeeding if PN). Intra-abdominal pressure (IAP)
Intra-abdominal infection	All previously described symptoms are possible Systemic signs of infection/sepsis	In other cases, if bowel continuity intact, GRV <500 mL and IAP <20 mmHg, start oral nutrition or gastric EN[a] [7]	Clinical assessment[a]. IAP Stool frequency, appearance, volume
Uncontrolled – (Retro)peritoneal bleeding – upper GI bleeding	– Hemodynamic instability. Increasing size of hemo(retro) peritoneum. Increasing IAP – Haematemesis, melaena. Hemodynamic instability	Endoscopic intervention, radiological intervention (coiling) or surgical management. No oral or enteral nutrition until active bleeding stopped and no signs of rebleeding within 24 h. Thereafter cautious oral diet or EN[b] [7]	Clinical assessment[a] Haemoglobin levels IAP

(continued)

TABLE 4.2 (continued)

Syndrome/ mechanism	Symptoms/consequences	Management strategy and nutritional implications	Monitoring
Acute (entero)colitis	Abdominal pain and distension Diarrhoea Systemic signs of infection/sepsis Colonic dilatation/distention Loss of fluids, electrolytes and nutrients	If severe bowel oedema along with severe bowel distension—delay EN for 24 h. Treat *C. difficile* infection. In other cases, if GRV <500 mL and IAP <20 mmHg, start EN with 10 mL/h and progress cautiously (e.g. 10 mL/h in 12–24 h). Supplemental PN after 4–7 days in case of insufficient EN or suspected malabsorption (cave overfeeding)	Clinical assessment[a] Stool frequency, appearance, volume IAP. Electrolytes Volume and acid-base status Signs of malabsorption
Severe acute pancreatitis	Vomiting, high GRV Abdominal distension and pain Elevated IAP (>12 mmHg) Retroperitoneal inflammation and necrosis aggravating hypomotility	Start gastric EN 10–20 mL/h if GRV <500 mL and IAP <20 mmHg If GRV >200 mL/6 h—see management of gastroparesis If ACS (IAP >20 mmHg + organ failure)—see management of ACS Consider replacement of pancreatic enzymes of elemental EN if pancreatic exocrine insufficiency suspected [13]	GRV IAP Faecal elastase-1 and faecal fat
Acute short bowel syndrome	Acute short bowel syndrome after (damage control) surgery with or without multiple stomata	Start oral or enteral nutrition with 20 mL/h. Increase by 10 mL/h 12-hourly if IAP and GRV are not increasing. Consider early (supplemental) PN if EN will be clearly insufficient for prolonged period or severe malabsorption is inevitable due to remaining bowel	Clinical assessment[a] Stool frequency, appearance, volume Skin lesions around stomata Electrolyte levels Signs of malabsorption

High-output stoma	A stoma with output of >1500 mL for 2 consecutive days is considered high-output stoma Loss of fluids, electrolytes and nutrients	Consider chyme reinfusion/enteroclysis if high-output proximal stoma with concomitant distal stoma/feeding access [3, 33]	Clinical assessment[a] Stool frequency, appearance, volume Skin lesions around stomata Electrolyte levels Signs of malabsorption
Intestinal fistula	Fistula output >500 mL is commonly considered high Loss of nutrients, digestive enzymes and fluids Loss of acid with proximal fistula	Aim feeding access distal to fistula. Consider octreotide [3]. Aim euvolemia If enteral access distal to fistula — EN. If high-output fistula, consider chyme reinfusion/fistuloclysis [3, 33]. Consider supplemental PN from day 4 *High-output fistula* without distal feeding access—no oral or EN [7]. Start PN. *Low-output fistula* without distal access—consider oral nutrition or EN proximal to fistula. Consider supplemental PN from day 4	Fistula output. Enteral losses Electrolyte levels, acid-base status Clinical assessment[a] Skin lesions around fistula

(continued)

Table 4.2 (continued)

Syndrome/ mechanism	Symptoms/consequences	Management strategy and nutritional implications	Monitoring
Anastomotic leakage/ internal fistula	Leakage of intestinal, pancreatic or biliary secretions in the abdomen Local inflammation Loss of digestive enzymes	Surgical re-anastomosis, stenting or drainage. Consider re-intervention if patient's general condition does not improve If enteral access distal to leakage—EN with supplementation of pancreatic enzymes or semi-elemental formula. Consider supplemental PN from day 4 Supplement electrolytes, vitamins and trace elements	Clinical assessment[a] Abdominal symptoms (local or diffuse) Volume and aspect of lost secretions Electrolyte levels

[a]Clinical assessment includes (1) signs of acute abdomen, (2) signs of bleeding and (3) signs of sepsis
[b]EN—see general precautions in Fig. 4.1

contents can prevent gastric distension. Distension of the stomach needs to be avoided, and therefore it is suggested to delay EN if GRV is >500 mL/6 h (Table 4.2) [7]. Importantly, frequency of measurements of GRV can be reduced once full EN is established and tolerated.

4.2.1.2   Paralytic Ileus

Paralytic ileus often occurs in the setting of systemic disease such as shock or sepsis or after surgery. Main underlying mechanisms include hypoperfusion and inflammation. Low-dose cautious EN can generally be initiated. However, paralytic ileus may be a sign of acute abdomen, which always needs to be excluded. A prerequisite for EN is that the bowel is well perfused, whereas presence of bowel sounds before starting EN is not necessary. An unpleasant frequent consequence of paralytic ileus is bowel distension.

4.2.1.3   Bowel Distension

Bowel distension occurs due to impaired bowel motility and excessive gas production by gut microflora. Bowel distension can be diagnosed by X-ray or CT scan and dynamically evaluated at the bedside by assessment of abdominal pain and distension.

4.2.1.4   Isolated Colonic Ileus and Ogilvie's Syndrome

Critical illness-related colonic ileus is characterized by the non-passage of stools for many days without marked colonic distension [8]. Time to first defecation may take a week and relates to severity of illness, vasoactive medication, administration of opioids and mechanical ventilation [9]. Colonic ileus may herald Ogilvie's syndrome manifesting in gross abdominal distension with tenderness most pronounced over the caecum. Gastroparesis is not necessarily present; bowel sounds are normal, diminished or high; and percussion is hypertympanic. If diagnosis and treatment are delayed, progressive distension may cause peritoneal signs, respiratory compromise, sepsis due to bacterial translocation, multiple organ failure, ischaemia and caecal perforation. The risk of perforation is unlikely, when caecal diameter is less than 12 cm, but increases sharply when caecal diameter is greater [10]. Prevention and timely radiological diagnosis are therefore crucial.

Colonic ileus requires a proactive strategy including administration of early oral laxatives (polyethylene glycol or lactulose) [8] and enemas, followed by a continuous infusion of neostigmine if defecation does not occur [11]. With this strategy, endoscopic or surgical decompression is seldom needed. Isolated colonic ileus is no reason to delay EN, unless peritoneal signs are present.

4.2.1.5   Diarrhoea

Diarrhoea frequently occurs in critically ill patients (14–21%) [12, 13] and may have variety of causes; differential diagnostics is therefore essential [13]. In patients with MODS, the main mechanisms leading to diarrhoea are hypoperfusion, use of antibiotics and opportunistic bacterial overgrowth. A recent observational study found that EN covering >60% of energy target was a risk factor next to the use of antibiotics or antifungal drugs [12]. Along with the diagnostic and therapeutic process, low-dose EN can be initiated and advanced cautiously. A recent meta-analysis showed that the addition of fibre to EN reduced diarrhoea in stable patients, but not in critically ill patients; prebiotics are not shown effective [14].

Patients with severe diarrhoea may lose substantial amounts of fluid, electrolytes and trace elements which should be supplemented intravenously. If diarrhoea originates from *maldigestion* or *malabsorption*, the uptake of nutrients will be diminished. Faecal examination may be useful to detect the loss of fat or fatty acids, whereas the presence of faecal elastase-1 suggests pancreatic insufficiency (see below), but respective data in critically ill are scarce. In the intensive care setting, enteral loss of protein can be due to lymphatic obstruction (due to bowel oedema, increased intra-abdominal and/or intrathoracic pressure) or mucosal disease (erosions, ulcerations, enteritis or colitis, graft-versus-host disease or cytomegalovirus reactivation). Severe hypoalbuminemia may develop.

4.2.1.6 Bowel Hypoperfusion and Intestinal Ischemia

The suspicion of intestinal hypoperfusion in presence of clinical deterioration, tense abdomen, increasing lactate and hemodynamic instability, suggests bowel ischaemia and gerenally requires laparotomy. If surgery is not indicated/performed, the adequacy of bowel perfusion is difficult to estimate. Bowel necrosis is frequently associated with hyperlactatemia, but precise cut-offs are not established. Bedside abdominal examination in ICU patients is often non-specific and non-conclusive. Therefore, in case of uncertainty, EN can be delayed with daily re-evaluation of the condition and started in a low dose if signs of ongoing bowel ischemia remain absent. Importantly, endoscopically detected ischemic lesions of bowel mucosa without clinical signs of transmural ischemia are no contraindication to trophic feeding. Speculatively, trophic feeding could even be protective as it may help restoring atrophic mucosa and stimulating bowel perfusion.

Importantly, abdominal aortic surgery results in colonic ischemia in about 2% of patients after elective surgery and in 10% after rupture of the aneurysm, somewhat less in endovascular repair [15]. Observations during surgery (e.g. large bowel viability, assessment of blood flow) and details of the surgical procedure (level of clamping, etc.) need to reach intensivist. Length of operation, aneurysm rupture and renal insufficiency have been identified as independent risk factors of colonic ischemia [15].

4.2.1.7   Intestinal Oedema

There are several mechanisms leading to intestinal oedema in critical illness: (1) fluid extravasation due to capillary leak, (2) decreased lymph flow due to impaired GI motility and increased intra-abdominal and/or intrathoracic pressures, (3) intra-abdominal hypertension (IAH) leading to venous congestion and splanchnic hypoperfusion and (4) right heart failure. Gut oedema increases the distance between cells and blood, thereby generating an additional physical barrier to absorption of nutrients and hindering oxygen transport. Fluid overload and associated oedema increase the risk of anastomotic leakage [16]. If severe bowel oedema is observed during surgery, especially if accompanied by bowel distension, delay of EN for 24 h can be considered.

4.2.1.8   Elevated Intra-abdominal Pressure

Abdominal compartment syndrome (ACS), defined as intra-abdominal Pressure (IAP) above 20 mmHg along with new or worsening organ failure [17], is an immediately life-threatening condition, where prompt measures to reduce IAP are needed. Therefore, EN should not be given to patients with ACS. Instead, gastric decompression should be performed along with other measures lowering intra-abdominal pressure. Intra-abdominal hypertension without abdominal compartment syndrome is not a contra-indication to EN, but EN seems to be less well tolerated when intra-abdominal pressure is increased [18]. A further increase in IAP under EN may necessitate stopping or reducing of EN [7].

4.2.1.9   Direct Injury/Lesion to the GI Tract

Direct injury to the GI tract is commonly associated with disturbed motility and local or generalized bowel oedema.

Major abdominal surgery or trauma may be associated with all previously described symptoms and pathophysiological mechanisms. Resection and re-anastomosis changes entero-enteral signalling leading to disturbed motility. Intestinal perfusion, presence of peritoneal contamination or infection, intestinal oedema and bowel distension need to be carefully evaluated during surgery, and it is crucial that this information is communicated to the intensivist along with details on surgical intervention.

Based on the kind of surgery, nutritional implications vary:

1. Oesophageal surgery commonly results in excision of the lower oesophageal sphincter and is therefore associated with disturbed upper GI motility and massively increased risk of aspiration. Therefore, early EN via stomach or duodenum should be avoided, whereas there is no contraindication for jejunal feeding. The surgeon should be encouraged to leave a jejunal tube during surgery distal from the anastomosis.

2. Bilio-/pancreatico-enteral anastomosis often causes some concern about EN stimulating pancreatic secretions and jeopardizing anastomosis healing. Results of randomized studies are controversial showing higher incidences of pancreatic fistula with jejunal versus parenteral nutrition in some [19] but also largely varying incidences of fistulisation, suggesting additional surgical factors [20]. Some of the fistulae may be related to the jejunal tube itself, causing mechanical damage or being positioned too close to the anastomosis.

3. Entero-enteral anastomosis is no reason to delay oral diet or EN unless performed on distended and oedematous bowel (see Sect. 4.2.1.7).

In general, early EN is considered beneficial after GI surgery, both elective and urgent [7].

Intra-abdominal or retroperitoneal bleeding that is managed conservatively requires monitoring of IAP and regular assessment via ultrasound, whereas low-dose EN can usually be started. Retroperitoneal hematoma often leads to IAH but additionally may cause hypomotility by impairing nerve conduction.

Ongoing or unresolved intra-abdominal infection is commonly causing hypomotility and hampering EN, but without presence of bowel leakage should not lead to delay in EN. However, all efforts to achieve source control are imperative. The presence of high GRVs, bowel paralysis and/or diarrhoea may indicate ongoing infection and trigger further diagnostics.

4.2.1.10   Acute (Entero)colitis

Acute colitis in critically ill patients is most commonly caused by *Clostridium difficile* infection with prevalence of up to 2% of admitted patients [9, 12, 21]. Consequences may be far-reaching due to nosocomial spread and potential escalation into severe pseudomembranous colitis. The most common risk factors are antibiotic use and prolonged hospital stay. *Neutropenic enterocolitis* is seen mainly in haematological patients receiving intense chemotherapy [22]. The caecum is always affected, but the neighbouring colon may also be involved. If the disease extends to the ileum, malabsorption may become prominent. Severe enterocolitis leads to paralysis and dilatation of the colon and is associated with disrupted mucosal surface, leading to intramural invasion and translocation of bacteria and fungi [23].

The presence of colitis is no contraindication for EN, but EN should be advanced cautiously. Full EN seems only to be justified if diarrhoea and abdominal symptoms do not worsen [12]. In refractory cases, especially in case of neutropenic colitis, (supplemental) parenteral nutrition (PN) may be inevitable, because recovery may take several weeks. Special attention should be paid to the monitoring and supplementation of electrolytes, trace elements and vitamins.

4.2.1.11   Pancreatic Pathology

Pancreatic exocrine insufficiency is thought to occur often during critically illness, whereas not only patients with known pancreatic disease are affected. Faecal elastase-1 concentration may be useful for diagnosis. Resulting maldigestion can be managed by the supplementation of pancreatic enzymes, but specific instructions for administration of these medications via feeding tubes need to be followed [24].

Acute Pancreatitis

Nutrition in severe acute pancreatitis is a challenge. In case of necrotizing pancreatitis, abdominal distension due to retro-peritoneal inflammation and necrosis is common, the extent depending on the severity of pancreatitis. Therefore, monitoring IAP is required. Multifactorial bowel paralysis (opioids, sedation, inflammation, local oedema) along with IAH may hinder EN, and protracted illness may necessitate supplemental PN. Still, EN should always be attempted unless acute pancrcatitis leads to abdominal compartment syndrome [7]. Nasogastric EN should be tried first using prokinetics in case of gastroparesis. However, a jejunal tube is often necessary. Duodenal EN is probably not optimal due to risk of tube dislocation into the stomach and possible stimulation of pancreatic secretions. Acute pancreatitis may be associated with exocrine insufficiency requiring supplementation of pancreatic enzymes.

4.2.2 Nutritional Strategy in AGI

Despite the large variety of conditions, nutritional strategy is quite similar (see details in Table 4.2 and Fig. 4.1). Despite GI dysfunction, the following hierarchy of routes for nutrition should still always be considered: (1) oral diet, (2) gastric EN, (3) jejunal EN and (4) PN. Not using the GI tract for nutrition requires a justification. Importantly, decisions to start oral diet or EN should not be based on presence or absence of bowel sounds. EN is always started in a low dose under monitoring of GI symptoms and increased only gradually. In all cases of AGI, avoidable causes of dysmotility (drugs, immobilization) should be addressed, and normalization of serum electrolyte levels is essential.

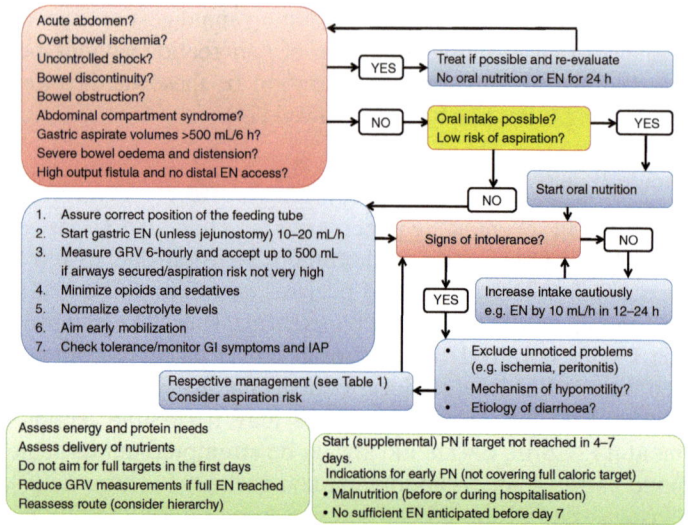

FIGURE 4.1 General nutritional strategy in patients with acute GI dysfunction/failure

Depending on the expected recovery time, (supplemental) PN should be initiated after 4–7 days [25–27]. Timing is based on the presence and duration of underfeeding before ICU admission and on expected recovery time (Fig. 4.1). A rapid increase of nutritional amounts may be harmful in patients with malnutrition because of refeeding and associated worse outcome [28]. Furthermore, nutrition (independent of route) covering full energy consumption is not the goal during the acute phase of illness and may even be unwanted as evidenced by several large trials showing similar [29, 30] or worse [26, 28] outcomes with full EN compared to trophic or hypocaloric nutrition. Overfeeding should at all times be avoided, and protein delivery should be adequate [31, 32].

4.3   Acute Protracted Intestinal Failure

4.3.1   Specific Characteristics

Intestinal failure as prolonged acute condition where absorptive capacity of the gut is reduced below the minimum needed for survival occurs very rarely [2, 3]. Examples of this category are acute short bowel syndrome, high-output fistula and high-output ileostoma. The associated large fluid shifts and electrolyte disturbances along with ongoing inflammation may result in other organ dysfunctions (e.g. renal or liver) and require temporary management in the ICU.

4.3.2   Nutritional Strategy

In case of acute prolonged intestinal failure (IF), EN may be impossible or insufficient for longer time periods if:

1. Surgery to achieve continuity of the GI tract is unsuccessful.
2. Short bowel syndrome does not allow achieving sufficient absorption of nutrients.
3. Enteral feeding intolerance persists due to bowel paralysis in prolonged intra-abdominal sepsis.

Understanding of the actual situation (which parts of the bowel are expected to be functional) and profound knowledge on the location of GI secretions and absorption of nutrients and fluids are required to identify maldigestion and malabsorption.

If sufficient EN is not anticipated within a week, (supplemental) PN should not be delayed [30]. In patients with a severe pre-admission caloric deficit, total caloric intake covering 100% of calculated/measured needs should be considered in the first days of ICU (re)admission if the severe acute condition (e.g. septic shock) has been stabilized. When signs of refeeding occur, a temporary reduction of feeding dose should be considered [29]. In most patients with short bowel syndrome, elemental feeding is not necessary, because secretion of digestive enzymes is adequate. However, (semi)elemental feeding may be considered in case of persisting diarrhoea with unclear cause [3] or loss of biliary and pancreatic secretions. Estimation of actual energy needs is especially difficult in these patients, and indirect calorimetry is the method of choice to define actual calorie needs. In case of (assumed) high protein losses, efforts to estimate and achieve adequate protein intake should be made [31, 32].

In case of high-output fistula or stoma, the collection of the proximal intestinal effluent and reinfusion of the chyme into the distal part of the intestine allow delivery of nutrients and digestive enzymes, which have trophic effects on the mucosa and may restore ileal brake [33].

Monitoring of nutrition intake, gastrointestinal losses, fluid and electrolyte status is important in all critically ill patients, but especially in patients with acute protracted IF. See Table 4.2. Special attention should be paid on the supplementation of vitamins and trace elements.

4.4   Summary

In patients with acute gastrointestinal dysfunction, EN should always be considered if oral intake is not feasible and bowel continuity is intact. EN should be delayed in case of uncontrolled upper GI bleeding, gastric aspirate >500 mL/6 h, bowel ischaemia, bowel obstruction, abdominal compartment syndrome and high-output fistula without distal feeding access. In most other patients with acute gastrointestinal injury, EN should be started in a low dose and increased slowly. In addition, measures to promote GI motility should be undertaken. Jejunal feeding should be considered if gastric aspirates and/or the risk of aspiration remain high. In most situations, PN should be started when EN is insufficient after 4–7 days but should be considered earlier in patients with a large pre-admission caloric deficit, paying special attention to refeeding syndrome and avoidance of overfeeding.

References

1. Reintam Blaser A, Malbrain ML, Starkopf J, Fruhwald S, Jakob SM, De Waele J, Braun JP, Poeze M, Spies C. Gastrointestinal function in intensive care patients: terminology, definitions and management. Recommendations of the ESICM Working Group on Abdominal Problems. Intensive Care Med. 2012;38(3):384–94.
2. Pironi L, Arends J, Baxter J, Bozzetti F, Peláez RB, Cuerda C, Forbes A, Gabe S, Gillanders L, Holst M, Jeppesen PB, Joly F, Kelly D, Klek S, Irtun Ø, Olde Damink SW, Panisic M, Rasmussen HH, Staun M, Szczepanek K, Van Gossum A, Wanten G, Schneider SM, Shaffer J, Home Artificial Nutrition & Chronic Intestinal Failure; Acute Intestinal Failure Special Interest Groups of ESPEN. ESPEN endorsed recommendations. Definition and classification of intestinal failure in adults. Clin Nutr. 2015;34(2):171–80.
3. Klek S, Forbes A, Gabe S, Holst M, Wanten G, Irtun Ø, Damink SO, Panisic-Sekeljic M, Pelaez RB, Pironi L, Reintam Blaser A, Rasmussen HH, Schneider SM, Thibault R, Visschers RG, Shaffer J. Management of acute intestinal failure: a position paper from the European Society for Clinical Nutrition and Metabolism (ESPEN) Special Interest Group. Clin Nutr. 2016;35(6):1209–18.
4. Reintam Blaser A, Jakob SM, Starkopf J. Gastrointestinal failure in the ICU. Curr Opin Crit Care. 2016;22(2):128–41.
5. Hamada SR, Garcon P, Ronot M, Kerever S, Paugam-Burtz C, Mantz J. Ultrasound assessment of gastric volume in critically ill patients. Intensive Care Med. 2014;40(7):965–72.
6. Reignier J, Mercier E, Le Gouge A, Boulain T, Desachy A, Bellec F, Clavel M, Frat JP, Plantefeve G, Quenot JP, Lascarrou JB. Clinical Research in Intensive Care and Sepsis (CRICS) Group. Effect of not monitoring residual gastric volume on risk of

ventilator-associated pneumonia in adults receiving mechanical ventilation and early enteral feeding: a randomized controlled trial. JAMA. 2013;309(3):249–56.

7. Reintam Blaser A, Starkopf J, Alhazzani W, Berger MM, Casaer MP, Deane AM, Fruhwald S, Hiesmayr M, Ichai C, Jakob SM, Loudet CI, Malbrain ML, Montejo González JC, Paugam-Burtz C, Poeze M, Preiser JC, Singer P, van Zanten AR, De Waele J, Wendon J, Wernerman J, Whitehouse T, Wilmer A, Oudemans-van Straaten HM. ESICM Working Group on Gastrointestinal Function. Early enteral nutrition in critically ill patients: ESICM clinical practice guidelines. Intensive Care Med. 2017;43(3):380–98.

8. van der Spoel JI, Oudemans-van Straaten HM, Kuiper MA, van Roon EN, Zandstra DF, van der Voort PH. Laxation of critically ill patients with lactulose or polyethylene glycol: a two-center randomized, double-blind, placebo-controlled trial. Crit Care Med. 2007;35(12):2726–31.

9. van der Spoel JI, Schultz MJ, van der Voort PH, de Jonge E. Influence of severity of illness, medication and selective decontamination on defecation. Intensive Care Med. 2006;32(6):875–80.

10. Saunders MD. Acute colonic pseudo-obstruction. Gastrointest Endosc Clin N Am. 2007;17(2):341–60.

11. van der Spoel JI, Oudemans-van Straaten HM, Stoutenbeek CP, Bosman RJ, Zandstra DF. Neostigmine resolves critical illness-related colonic ileus in intensive care patients with multiple organ failure—a prospective, double-blind, placebo-controlled trial. Intensive Care Med. 2001;27(5):822–7.

12. Thibault R, Graf S, Clerc A, Delieuvin N, Heidegger CP, Pichard C. Diarrhoea in the ICU: respective contribution of feeding and antibiotics. Crit Care. 2013;17:R153.

13. Reintam Blaser A, Deane AM, Fruhwald S. Diarrhoea in the critically ill. Curr Opin Crit Care. 2015;21(2):142–53.

14. Kamarul Zaman M, Chin KF, Rai V, Majid HA. Fiber and prebiotic supplementation in enteral nutrition: a systematic review and meta-analysis. World J Gastroenterol. 2015;21(17): 5372–81.

15. Becquemin JP1, Majewski M, Fermani N, Marzelle J, Desgrandes P, Allaire E, Roudot-Thoraval F. Colon ischemia following abdominal aortic aneurysm repair in the era of endovascular

abdominal aortic repair. J Vasc Surg. 2008;47(2):258–63; discussion 263.

16. Nessim C, Sidéris L, Turcotte S, Vafiadis P, Lapostole AC, Simard S, Koch P, Fortier LP, Dubé P. The effect of fluid overload in the presence of an epidural on the strength of colonic anastomoses. J Surg Res. 2013;183(2):567–73.

17. Kirkpatrick AW, Roberts DJ, De Waele J, Jaeschke R, Malbrain ML, De Keulenaer B, Duchesne J, Bjorck M, Leppaniemi A, Ejike JC, Sugrue M, Cheatham M, Ivatury R, Ball CG, Reintam Blaser A, Regli A, Balogh ZJ, D'Amours S, Debergh D, Kaplan M, Kimball E, Olvera C, Pediatric Guidelines Sub-Committee for the World Society of the Abdominal Compartment Syndrome. Intra-abdominal hypertension and the abdominal compartment syndrome: updated consensus definitions and clinical practice guidelines from the World Society of the Abdominal Compartment Syndrome. Intensive Care Med. 2013;39(7):1190–206.

18. Bejarano N, Navarro S, Rebasa P, García-Esquirol O, Hermoso J. Intra-abdominal pressure as a prognostic factor for tolerance of enteral nutrition in critical patients. JPEN J Parenter Enteral Nutr. 2013;37(3):352–60.

19. Perinel J, Mariette C, Dousset B, et al. Early enteral versus total parenteral nutrition in patients undergoing pancreaticoduodenectomy: a randomized multicenter controlled trial (Nutri-DPC). Ann Surg. 2016;264:731–7.

20. Cereda E, Caccialanza R, Pedrolli C. Feeding after pancreaticoduodenectomy: enteral, or parenteral, that is the question. J Thorac Dis. 2016;8(11):E1478–80.

21. Karanika S, Paudel S, Zervou FN, Grigoras C, Zacharioudakis IM, Mylonakis E. Prevalence and clinical outcomes of *Clostridium difficile* infection in the intensive care unit: a systematic review and meta-analysis. Open Forum Infect Dis. 2015;3(1):ofv186. eCollection 2016.

22. Rodrigues FG, Dasilva G, Wexner SD. Neutropenic enterocolitis. World J Gastroenterol. 2017;23(1):42–7.

23. Lebon D, Biard L, Buyse S, Schnell D, Lengliné E, Roussel C, Gornet JM, Munoz-Bongrand N, Quéro L, Resche-Rigon M, Azoulay E, Canet E. Gastrointestinal emergencies in critically ill cancer patients. J Crit Care. 2017;40:69–75.

24. Ferrie S, Graham C, Hoyle M. Pancreatic enzyme supplementation for patients receiving enteral feeds. Nutr Clin Pract. 2011;26(3):349–51.
25. Heidegger CP, Berger MM, Graf S, Zingg W, Darmon P, Costanza MC, Thibault R, Pichard C. Optimisation of energy provision with supplemental parenteral nutrition in critically ill patients: a randomised controlled clinical trial. Lancet. 2013;381(9864):385–93.
26. Casaer MP, Mesotten D, Hermans G, Wouters PJ, Schetz M, Meyfroidt G, Van Cromphaut S, Ingels C, Meersseman P, Muller J, Vlasselaers D, Debaveye Y, Desmet L, Dubois J, Van Assche A, Vanderheyden S, Wilmer A, Van den Berghe G. Early versus late parenteral nutrition in critically ill adults. N Engl J Med. 2011;365(6):506–17.
27. Doig GS, Simpson F, Sweetman EA, Finfer SR, Cooper DJ, Heighes PT, et al. Early parenteral nutrition in critically ill patients with short-term relative contraindications to early enteral nutrition: a randomized controlled trial. JAMA. 2013;309:2130–8.
28. Doig GS, Simpson F, Heighes PT, Bellomo R, Chesher D, Caterson ID, Reade MC, Harrigan PW. Refeeding Syndrome Trial Investigators Group. Restricted versus continued standard caloric intake during the management of refeeding syndrome in critically ill adults: a randomised, parallel-group, multicentre, single-blind controlled trial. Lancet Respir Med. 2015;3(12):943–52.
29. National Heart, Lung, and Blood Institute Acute Respiratory Distress Syndrome (ARDS) Clinical Trials Network, Rice TW, Wheeler AP, Thompson BT, Steingrub J, Hite RD, Moss M, Morris A, Dong N, Rock P. Initial trophic vs full enteral feeding in patients with acute lung injury: the EDEN randomized trial. JAMA. 2012;307(8):795–803.
30. Arabi YM, Aldawood AS, Haddad SH, Al-Dorzi HM, Tamim HM, Jones G, Mehta S, McIntyre L, Solaiman O, Sakkijha MH, Sadat M, Afesh L, Permit Trial Group. Permissive underfeeding or standard enteral feeding in critically ill adults. N Engl J Med. 2015;372(25):2398–408.
31. Weijs PJ, Looijaard WG, Beishuizen A, Girbes AR, Oudemans-van Straaten HM. Early high protein intake is associated with

low mortality and energy overfeeding with high mortality in non-septic mechanically ventilated critically ill patients. Crit Care. 2014;18(6):701.

32. Zusman O, Theilla M, Cohen J, Kagan I, Bendavid I, Singer P. Resting energy expenditure, calorie and protein consumption in critically ill patients: a retrospective cohort study. Crit Care. 2016;20(1):367.

33. Thibault R, Picot D. Chyme reinfusion or enteroclysis in nutrition of patients with temporary double enterostomy or enterocutaneous fistula. Curr Opin Clin Nutr Metab Care. 2016;19(5):382–87.

.

Chapter 5
Brain Injury and Nutrition

Hervé Quintard and Carole Ichai

The benefits of nutritional support in critical illness are widely accepted and supported by objective reviews. Traumatic brain injury (TBI) is a significant public health concern. Limited provision of metabolic support to neurotrauma has been underlined [1]. Nutritional status is associated with the length of mechanical ventilation and time until discharge from ICU or hospital [2]. There is a need for developing evidence-based interventions to reduce the morbidity. A better understanding on metabolic rate, caloric and macronutrients requirements, on mechanisms involved in enteral feeding intolerance is essential to improve nutrition in this setting. The purpose of this chapter is to expose an overview of the management of nutritional support in neuro intensive care unit (NICU) patients.

H. Quintard, M.D., Ph.D. (✉)
Intensive Care Unit, Pasteur 2 Hospital,
30 Voie Romaine, CNRS UMR 7275, 06001 Nice, Cédex 1, France
e-mail: quintard.h@chu-nice.fr

C. Ichai
University Hospital of Nice, Intensive Care Unit, Pasteur 2
Hospital, 30 Voie Romaine, IRCAN (INSERM U1081, CNRS
UMR 7284), 06001 Nice, Cédex 1, France

© Springer International Publishing AG 2018   67
M.M. Berger (ed.), *Critical Care Nutrition Therapy
for Non-nutritionists*, https://doi.org/10.1007/978-3-319-58652-6_5

5.1   Metabolic Rate and Macronutrient Needs

Neurological injuries induce a cascade of sympathetic nervous system activation and inflammatory response resulting in a well-described hypermetabolic response [3]. Several studies mostly in TBI patients have been conducted using indirect calorimetry (IDC), the gold standard method to assess resting energy expenditure (REE) after brain injury [4]. REE increased after TBI and may vary from 75 to 200% in two-thirds of patients during the first 2–4 weeks following trauma [4, 5]. This hypermetabolic state has been described in other cerebrovascular diseases such as stroke [6]. However, the studies failed to identify the best timing, duration, and frequency to assess REE. The metabolic rate among brain-injured patients is summarized in Table 5.1 [6]. Observational data confirm that critically TBI patients are substantially underfed. In patients with moderate to severe TBI, the mean cumulative energy deficit estimated as the difference between support and estimated requirements, according Schofield equation in ICU, was evaluated to 18.2 kcal and persisted over the hospitalization [7]. Few studies using IDC assessing the real requirement in this setting are reported in the literature.

The nitrogen balance is the only biomarker for protein energy metabolism, widely reported in the neurocritical care population. Randomized control trials (RCTs) measuring nitrogen balance or the degree of nitrogen loss have been performed and suggest that less than 50% of administered nitrogen is retained after TBI. The non-accordance between supply and need is associated with a poor prognosis, an increased in-hospital, in-ICU length of stay, and an increased length of mechanical ventilation [2]. In practice, it is recommended to provide *20–25 kcal/kg of actual body weight (BW) per day* during the acute phase and reach 25–30 kcal/kg BW per day in the stable phase.

TABLE 5.1 Variation of metabolic rate (indirect calorimetry) according to brain injury type and level of sedation [6]

Resting metabolic rate (kcal/day)			
	Sedated	Not sedated	All
Ischemic stroke	1903 ± 205	1954 ± 203	1929 ± 205
Hemorrhagic stroke	2076 ± 198	1937 ± 201	2007 ± 208
Traumatic brain injury	1915 ± 199	2187 ± 202	2051 ± 220

Results express as mean ± SD

Numerous factors contribute to modify REE in TBI patients: temperature, sedation, paralyzing agents, mechanical ventilation, barbiturates, and the severity of trauma. Sedation is responsible for a 10–30% reduction in basal energy expenditure (BEE) [6]. Most authors consider that TBI's energy expenditure is 1.4 of BEE and 1 of BEE in case of sedation and muscular blockade use, respectively. Hyperthermia which is more frequently present in most severe TBI is also associated with a higher energy expenditure. Therefore, large variations in energy expenditure are observed in TBI, and the estimation of caloric requirements is difficult. The protein caloric contribution is usually less than 20% and can increase to 30% in the acute phase of cerebrovascular disease. The intensive administration of protein preparation is necessary. Experts propose to supply *1–2 g/kg of BW per day* corresponding to 15% of the energy supply [5, 8].

Hyperglycemia (>11 mmol/L) has been largely reported to be associated with a worse outcome in observational studies performed in TBI [9, 10]. Glucose intakes should be controlled in order to avoid severe hyperglycemia and hypoglycemia which are both deleterious on brain and spinal cord injury. Strict control of glycemia with intensive insulinotherapy was found to be associated with an increased cerebral energetic crisis (elevated intracerebral lactate/ pyruvate ratio and glutamate) and a decreased cerebral glucose concentration (Table 5.2) [11]. Moreover, this strategy increases the risk of hypoglycemia. A recent trial has reported a poor relationship in brain-injured patient, between intra-arterial glucose and intracerebral glucose measured with microdialysis [12]. This emphasizes the potential benefit of using microdialysis to prevent cerebral hypoglycemia. Finally, recent randomized controlled trials and meta-analysis showed that glycemic control aiming to maintain glucose plasma level between 150 and 200 mg/dL failed to increase both mortality rate and poor outcome while reducing hypoglycemic episodes compared with a "strict glycemic control" [13]. Therefore, it is now recommended to avoid excessive hyperglycemia, i.e., >10–11 mmol/L (180–200 mg/dL) and to maintain a moderate "permissive" glycemic control *between 8 and 11 mmol/L (140–200 mg/dL)* [14]. Arterial blood glucose is the gold standard sampling site for measuring and monitoring glycemia. The rate of control is directly driven according to the *insulin therapy* (each 1–4 h). Carbohydrate supply as a part of nutrition in TBI should be *≤150 g/day* [15].

Most of patient in NICU are sedated with propofol which can deliver a high level of lipid [16]. Recommendation on lipid intake has been proposed to not exceed 1.5 g/kg/day for patients in ICU [17]. The available data are insufficient to support such a recommendation in NICU.

Despite abundant experimental evidence, the role of n-3 polyunsaturated fatty acid (n-3 PUFA) dietary supplementation in patients is not proven [18, 19]. Therefore, we cannot recommend, presently, such systematic supplementation in clinical practice.

TABLE 5.2 Clinical guidelines in brain injured patient

• Indirect calorimetry remains the gold standard to assess nutritional requirements in brain injury. If not available, we suggest to use predictive equation or to target a support of 20–25 kcal/kg of actual body weight (BW) per day during the acute phase and reach 25–30 kcal/kg BW per day in the stable phase

• Start enteral nutrition as soon as possible when patient is hemodynamically stable

• Prefer enteral nutrition to parenteral if possible

• Gastric residual volume measurement, enable detecting pyloric dysfunction during feeding initiation but must not be systematically monitored

• Gastric intolerance must be treated using metoclopramide. Prophylactic treatment is not recommended

• Continuous nutritional feeding may require use of prokinetics

• Glucose control to maintain normoglycemia, measured with arterial blood sample, between 8 and 11 mol/L is based on insulin treatment and monitored each 1–4 h

• Glycemia <3.3 mmol/L is defined as a hypoglycemic episode requiring glucose supplementation

• Cerebral glucose <1 mmol/L or lactate-on-pyruvate ratio >25 in microdialysis measurement has to conduct to control glycemia (insulin treatment or glucose supply)

• Intravenous Glutamine (0.3–0.5 g/kg) can be proposed in brain-injured patient

• Despite the absence of strong evidence, the parenteral supplementation of Zinc (12 mg) for 15 days in severe brain injured patient and/or vitamin D (200 UI/kg for 5 days) could be added to nutritional support

5.2   Implementation of Nutrition in Brain-Injured Patient

Observational studies show that brain-injured patients receive only 50% of the energy and protein requirement during their hospitalization [20]. Several reasons can explain this phenomenon [21]. Firstly, 50% of TBI patients exhibit intolerance to enteral nutrition, with a significantly prolonged gastric emptying: this disturbance may persist for the first 7–15 days following trauma [22]. Secondly, repetitive interruptions of enteral nutrition are quite frequent due to several constraints such as surgery and imaging exams. Enteral nutrition in TBI was stopped in 63% of days in ICU [2]. Recommendations concerning the use of prokinetics remain controversial: metoclopramide as the first treatment for the ASPEN-SCCM [8] while erythromycin is not recommended by ESPEN [17]. The jejunal route might be used in case of gastric hypokinesia despite appropriate strategies. Two meta-analysis failed to demonstrate any difference between the enteral and the parenteral route of feeding [1, 23]. However, considering potential beneficial effects of enteral route including immunologic response, gut integrity (trophic advantages), and lower cost, the ASPEN-SCCM suggests to prefer the enteral route of feeding in TBI when possible [8]. Enteral feeding should be initiated early, within 24–48 h of injury, once the patient is hemodynamically stable [8] even no data allows to determine the most precise appropriate timing. Enteral feeding must be gradually increased to reach at least 50% of the caloric and protein targets at day 3–5. If these objectives are not reached, supplemental parenteral nutrition must be initiated at day 3–5 and in all cases before day 7. When enteral nutrition is totally contraindicated, total parenteral nutrition is required in the same delay.

Feeding supplementation can be proposed in TBI patient. *Glutamine*-enriched enteral diets (0.3–0.5 g/kg BW), could reduce in-hospital length of stay, and infections in moderate to severe TBI patients. A zinc and vitamin D deficiency occurred in TBI patient because of an increased urinary excretion and a reduced bioavailability. These nutrients might improve neurologic outcome and reduce cerebral inflammation [24]. Despite the absence of strong evidence, the parenteral supplementation by zinc (12 mg) for 15 days in patients severely brain injured and/or vitamin D (200 UI/kg) for 5 days could be added to nutritional support.

5.3   Conclusion

Brain-injured patients present a hypermetabolism characterized by an elevated energy expenditure and protein loss. Inadequate nutritional support is directly associated with the worsening of prognosis. Particular attention to intolerance to enteral nutrition is essential to improve calories delivery. Early enteral feeding with high-protein polymeric diet should be initiated within the 24–48 h after injury, once the patient is hemodynamically stable. The accurate evaluation of metabolism of brain-injured patients remains difficult, and a nutritional support of 25 kcal/kg/day with 1.3–2 g/kg/day of protein at the acute phase is strongly suggested. A progressive increased enteral nutrition is preferred to parenteral nutrition, which may be proposed as rescue feeding. To assume adequate supplementation, formalized protocol including caloric requirements, procedures to improve nutritional support, have to be developed. Immunonutrition, with glutamine, vitamin D, and zinc, might find an interesting place in this group of patients, as seem to be associated with an improved prognosis.

References

1. Wang X, Dong Y, Han X, Qi X-Q, Huang C-G, Hou L-J. Nutritional support for patients sustaining traumatic brain injury: a systematic review and meta-analysis of prospective studies. PLoS One. 2013;8(3):e58838.
2. Chapple L-AS, Chapman MJ, Lange K, Deane AM, Heyland DK. Nutrition support practices in critically ill head-injured patients: a global perspective. Crit Care Lond Engl. 2016;20:6.
3. Clifton GL, Robertson CS, Choi SC. Assessment of nutritional requirements of head-injured patients. J Neurosurg. 1986;64(6):895–901.
4. Krakau K, Hansson A, Karlsson T, de Boussard CN, Tengvar C, Borg J. Nutritional treatment of patients with severe traumatic brain injury during the first six months after injury. Nutr Burbank Los Angel Cty Calif. 2007;23(4):308–17.
5. Foley N, Marshall S, Pikul J, Salter K, Teasell R. Hypermetabolism following moderate to severe traumatic acute brain injury: a systematic review. J Neurotrauma. 2008;25(12):1415–31.
6. Frankenfield DC, Ashcraft CM. Description and prediction of resting metabolic rate after stroke and traumatic brain injury. Nutr Burbank Los Angel Cty Calif. 2012;28(9):906–11.
7. Chapple L-AS, Deane AM, Heyland DK, Lange K, Kranz AJ, Williams LT, et al. Energy and protein deficits throughout hospitalization in patients admitted with a traumatic brain injury. Clin Nutr Edinb Scotl. 2016;35(6):1315–22.
8. Taylor BE, McClave SA, Martindale RG, Warren MM, Johnson DR, Braunschweig C, et al. Guidelines for the provision and assessment of nutrition support therapy in the adult critically ill patient: Society of Critical Care Medicine (SCCM) and American Society for Parenteral and Enteral Nutrition (A.S.P.E.N.). Crit Care Med. 2016;44(2):390–438.
9. Matsushima K, Peng M, Velasco C, Schaefer E, Diaz-Arrastia R, Frankel H. Glucose variability negatively impacts long-term functional outcome in patients with traumatic brain injury. J Crit Care. 2012;27(2):125–31.
10. Diaz-Parejo P, Ståhl N, Xu W, Reinstrup P, Ungerstedt U, Nordström C-H. Cerebral energy metabolism during transient hyperglycemia in patients with severe brain trauma. Intensive Care Med. 2003;29(4):544–50.

11. Vespa P, Mcarthur DL, Stein N, Huang S-C, Shao W, Filippou M, et al. Tight glycemic control increases metabolic distress in traumatic brain injury: a randomized controlled within-subjects trial. Crit Care Med. 2012;40(6):1923–9.

12. Rostami E, Bellander B-M. Monitoring of glucose in brain, adipose tissue, and peripheral blood in patients with traumatic brain injury: a microdialysis study. J Diabetes Sci Technol. 2011;5(3):596–604.

13. NICE-SUGAR Study Investigators for the Australian and New Zealand Intensive Care Society Clinical Trials Group and the Canadian Critical Care Trials Group, Finfer S, Chittock D, Li Y, Foster D, Dhingra V, et al. Intensive versus conventional glucose control in critically ill patients with traumatic brain injury: long-term follow-up of a subgroup of patients from the NICE-SUGAR study. Intensive Care Med. 2015;41(6):1037–47.

14. Oddo M, Schmidt JM, Carrera E, Badjatia N, Connolly ES, Presciutti M, et al. Impact of tight glycemic control on cerebral glucose metabolism after severe brain injury: a microdialysis study. Crit Care Med. 2008;36(12):3233–8.

15. Wolfe RR, Allsop JR, Burke JF. Glucose metabolism in man: responses to intravenous glucose infusion. Metabolism. 1979;28(3):210–20.

16. Devaud J-C, Berger MM, Pannatier A, Marques-Vidal P, Tappy L, Rodondi N, et al. Hypertriglyceridemia: a potential side effect of propofol sedation in critical illness. Intensive Care Med. 2012;38(12):1990–8.

17. Singer P, Berger MM, Van den Berghe G, Biolo G, Calder P, Forbes A, et al. ESPEN guidelines on parenteral nutrition: intensive care. Clin Nutr Edinb Scotl. 2009;28(4):387–400.

18. Lin C, Chao H, Li Z, Xu X, Liu Y, Bao Z, et al. Omega-3 fatty acids regulate NLRP3 inflammasome activation and prevent behavior deficits after traumatic brain injury. Exp Neurol. 2017;290:115–22.

19. Lewis MD. Concussions, traumatic brain injury, and the innovative use of omega-3s. J Am Coll Nutr. 2016;35(5):469–75.

20. Cahill NE, Dhaliwal R, Day AG, Jiang X, Heyland DK. Nutrition therapy in the critical care setting: what is "best achievable" practice? An international multicenter observational study. Crit Care Med. 2010;38(2):395–401.

21. Tan M, Zhu J-C, Yin H-H. Enteral nutrition in patients with severe traumatic brain injury: reasons for intolerance and medical management. Br J Neurosurg. 2011;25(1):2–8.

22. Kao CH, ChangLai SP, Chieng PU, Yen TC. Gastric emptying in head-injured patients. Am J Gastroenterol. 1998;93(7):1108–12.
23. Perel P, Yanagawa T, Bunn F, Roberts I, Wentz R, Pierro A. Nutritional support for head-injured patients. Cochrane Database Syst Rev. 2006;(4):CD001530.
24. Young B, Ott L, Kasarskis E, Rapp R, Moles K, Dempsey RJ, et al. Zinc supplementation is associated with improved neurologic recovery rate and visceral protein levels of patients with severe closed head injury. J Neurotrauma. 1996;13(1):25–34.

Chapter 6
Major Burns

Olivier Pantet and Mette M. Berger

6.1 Introduction

Among critically ill patients, the patients admitted for major burn injuries (i.e., involving more than 20% of body surface) have several specificities that differentiate them from non-burn patients and modulate their nutritional requirements. Table 6.1 summarizes the most significant differences. The inflammatory response elicited by the injury is among the most intense and prolonged that can be observed in the ICU and contributes to complications including multiple organ failure [1]. Herndon and Tompkins stated in 2004 that "The effective anabolic strategies for severe burn injuries are early excision and grafting of the wound; prompt treatment of sepsis, maintenance of environmental temperature at 30–32 °C, continuous feeding of a high carbohydrate, high protein diet, preferably by the enteral route, and early institution of vigorous and aerobic resistive exercise programs" [2]. This remains true more than a decade later despite the inclusion in the strategy of pharmacological modulation of catabolism and

O. Pantet (✉) • M.M. Berger
Service of adult Intensive care Medicine and Burns, Lausanne University Hospital (CHUV), Lausanne 1011, Switzerland
e-mail: Olivier.Pantet@chuv.ch

© Springer International Publishing AG 2018   77
M.M. Berger (ed.), *Critical Care Nutrition Therapy for Non-nutritionists*, https://doi.org/10.1007/978-3-319-58652-6_6

Table 6.1 Clinical and metabolic characteristics of major burn patients

	Changes	Consequences	References
Skin destruction	Loss of barrier function	Exudative fluid and mineral losses	[22]
		Wound repair	
Inflammation	Massive acute phase response	Massive cytokine release	[23]
Immune depression	Depressions of humoral and cellular immunity	Elevated infectious risk	[24]
Endocrine stress response	Initial intense stress response followed by depression of the hypothalamic-pituitary-adrenal axis – Low T3 syndrome – Sexual hormone depression	Long-term alterations with multiple changes – T3 levels (very low), testosterone in males (very low), LH is reported to be low – Unusually low (T4, FSH, androstenedione, progesterone—the latter especially in females) – High: dehydroepiandrosterone (DHEA), ADH, catecholamine, renin and angiotensin II, cortisolUsually elevated, but not always (ACTH, aldosterone, prolactin, glucagon insulin, beta-endorphin, reverse T3, 11-beta-hydroxyandrostenedione) –TSH is usually normal	[7]

TABLE 6.1 (continued)

	Changes	Consequences	References
Energy metabolism	Ebb and flow phases	Initial depression (ebb phase)	[2, 5]
		Increase (flow phase) is variable over time being the most pronounced during the first 2–4 weeks depending on burn size	
Nutritional requirements	Strongly increased	Protein requirements much superior to other non-burn conditions	[5]
		Increase affects all substrates and micronutrients	
Bone metabolism	Prolonged bedridden period	Hypercalcemia, demineralization, osteoporosis	[17]

anabolism. Indeed despite advances in treatment strategies, this exacerbated response and the associated hypermetabolism and catabolism persist [3] and require a sustained effort during the ICU stay. Hypermetabolism has recently been thought to result from an uncoupling of mitochondrial respiration from ADP phosphorylation resulting in heat production deeply affecting metabolism [4].

Major burn injury is probably the pathology in which nutrition therapy has been most convincingly shown to be part of the overall ICU therapy and heavily contribute to outcome. Its aim can be summarized as a combination of strategies that blunt the hypermetabolic response (up to twice the normal, lasting more than 1 year) and its consequences in conjunction with the other ICU therapies: this role starts already during the resuscitation phase, with the very early introduction of enteral feeding. The present text aims at providing daily practical guidance based on the most recent guidelines [5].

6.2   Specific Metabolic and Nutritional Characteristics

The destruction of the skin results in a series of specific problems: loss of the thermal isolation barrier, exudative losses of fluids and micronutrients defenses proportional to the size of the injury [6], and loss of the anti-infectious barrier. In addition, the amount of tissue requiring repair is very large varying between 0.5 and 2 m^2 of the skin. The inflammatory, endocrine, and metabolic responses, although much larger than in other pathologies, follow similar patterns and have been reviewed by others [7].

After major burn, an overwhelming endocrine storm affects all metabolic pathways with the release of massive quantities of stress hormones. A depression of the pituitary-adrenal, pituitary-gonadal, and pituitary-thyroid axes follows: the patients are characterized by a severe deficit of growth hormone and sexual hormones that lasts at least 2 months, in the most severely injured patients [8].

6.3   Timing of Nutritional Intervention

The gastrointestinal tract suffers from the intense stress response with massive catecholamine release and the fluid shifts caused by the capillary leak and required fluid resuscitation. Curling stress ulcers were first described in major burns. The early use of the gut improves blood flow to the gut, preserves the intestinal mucosal integrity, and attenuates the endocrine stress response. Oxidative stress being intense, a reinforcement of endogenous micronutrient defenses is associated with an attenuation of the deleterious effects. An early nutritional support (<24 h) is therefore recommended [5, 9].

6.4   Feeding Route

Enteral nutrition (EN) has repeatedly been shown to be the optimal feeding route in burns [5]: it rarely fails if initiated early, by preventing the ileus from resuscitation edema that would paralyze the gut after about 48 h of "nonuse." The beneficial effects of EN are maintenance of intestinal motility, attenuation of the endocrine stress response, improved immunity, and reduction of infectious complications. Post-pyloric tubes should be considered early in case of post-burn ileus and in those patients with massive burns who require nearly daily procedures under anesthesia, as the post-pyloric placement enables shortening the fasting time before and after anesthesia. Parenteral nutrition must be considered as a rescue therapy. The oral route has no role during the initial resuscitation phase, as oral intakes are not expected to meet the high caloric demand.

6.4.1   Energy Requirements

After the shock phase also called ebb phase, which is hypometabolic, a hypermetabolic phase called flow phase appears already after 2–3 days in association with the inflammatory response. Indirect calorimetry is ideally used to determine feeding target (measured energy expenditure is considered to be the target). When unavailable, the Toronto equation is a good option [5]. Other formulas such as the Curreri formula overestimate metabolic requirements and do not integrate the changing energy expenditure (EE) over time: they should be abandoned. A regular reevaluation, ideally by measurement of the EE, is mandatory, since it will vary greatly during the hospital stay. A careful monitoring of the caloric intake, with the help of a patient data management system (PDMS), can help avoiding both under- and overfeeding, by taking into account nonnutritive calories such as those included in propofol or dextrose solutions. Alternatively, Excel files can assist this monitoring. On the other hand, burned patients must be screened for underfeeding, as they are frequently fasted for surgery.

6.5   Specific Needs in Major Burns

6.5.1   Proteins

A severe proteolysis is a constant finding in major burn patients. The first studies challenging the protein requirements were carried out in burned children in the 1980s, showing that the administration of 2 g/kg was associated with a better outcome [2]. The catabolic response observed after major burns can be life threatening. Its intensity will depend on the magnitude of the inflammatory response and can only partially be attenuated by feeding which allows a reduction of negative nitrogen balance [10]. Increasing the protein intake may not be sufficient; a quality control study in adults recently confirmed that despite an increased protein intake, a reduction of energy intake worsens outcome and is associated with greater weight loss [11]. Protein requirement are currently estimated to be 1.5–2.0 g/kg/day for adult and 1.5–3.0 g/kg/day for children [5].

6.5.2   Glutamine

Major burn is (with trauma) the condition for which a level A grade of evidence supports the administration of enteral glutamine [5]. This amino acid is called "conditionally essential" as circulating and tissue glutamine concentrations decrease massively following large burns. Several randomized supplementation trials in burn patients have shown reduced mortality and decreased infectious complications [12]. Suggested doses are 0.3–0.5 g/kg/day during 10 days or more, according to extent of burn injury, as increased requirements are related to open burn wounds.

6.5.3   Glucose

Based on stable isotope studies [13], it is recommended to deliver as much as 60% of energy as carbohydrates to cover the energy needs of the rapidly proliferating glucose-dependent cells, but not to exceed this proportion. However, the threshold of 5 mg/kg/min (i.e. 7 g/kg/day) should not be exceeded. Insulin resistance is present from the start. Despite the risk of hypoglycemia, intensive insulin therapy is both safe and beneficial [2, 14]. The blood glucose to be aimed is therefore 6–10 mmol/L as for general ICU patients.

6.5.4   Trace Elements

Due to their large cutaneous exudative losses, the major burn patients develop an early acute and prolonged trace element (TE) deficiency condition affecting particularly copper (Cu), selenium (Se), and zinc (Zn). These losses stop with wound closure. The repletion requirements are therefore determined by the burned surface: 5–7 days for burns 20–40%, 2 weeks for burns 40–60%, and 30 days for burns >60% TBSA. As an example, our TE cocktail consist in Cu 3.75 mg, Se 0.17 mg, and Zn 30 mg combined to a daily parenteral nutrition dose of other elements. Plasma levels should be monitored regularly, probably weekly. Beware of patients undergoing CRRT as they need higher repletion doses.

6.5.5   Vitamins

High-dose vitamin C (66 mg/kg/h) during the first 24 h has been shown to reduce the initial fluid resuscitation requirements, by preventing the loosening of the intercellular tight junction, although definitive proofs are needed [15]. Vitamin C requirements are elevated through the wound healing period: 0.5–1.0 g/day is considered a standard intake.

Burn patients are particularly prone to vitamin D deficiency for multiple reasons. Dietary intakes of vitamin D are insufficient to correct plasma levels in burned patients [16]. Vitamin D repletion could reduce the risk of development of osteoporosis and the risk of fracture [17] or even muscular strength [18] as illustrated in pediatric studies, although the exact repletion dose is not known.

6.5.6   Anti-catabolic and Anabolic Agents and Other Tools

Beta-blockade with propranolol has become a standard since the Galveston randomized trial, which showed that catabolism was significantly attenuated in children [2].

Further, oxandrolone administration has been shown to exert major beneficial effects on both lean body mass but also in the prevention of osteoporosis, promoting the recovery of bone mass [19], these results being confirmed in a meta-analysis of 15 trials [20].

Finally, administration of recombinant growth hormone has been shown to result in positive biological effects in children but not in adults: despite this potential, it cannot be considered a standard treatment [5].

Non-nutritional measures should not be forgotten and include early excision of necrotic tissue and grafting, nursing in warm surrounding, and early mobilization.

6.6   Monitoring

As other critically ill patients, the burn patients receive less enteral feeding than what they are prescribed [21]. Monitoring real energy and protein delivery is of particular importance [11]. The monitoring of their nutrition therapy therefore is similar to that of other critically ill patients with the addition of a few specificities: plasma TE (Cu, Se, Zn) weekly in patients with burns >30%, response to protein intake, and more frequent determination of the actual weight. (see Chap. 1, Fig. 1.3, which summarizes general monitoring).

6.7   Conclusion

Major burns require particular attention to their nutrition therapy: massive catabolism persists long into the recovery phase and mandates particular attention to the protein intake. Energy requirements need adaptation over time. The paradox is that the nutrition therapy can be even better standardized as other critically ill.

References

1. Moore FA, Phillips SM, McClain CJ, Patel JJ, Martindale RG. Nutrition support for persistent inflammation, immunosuppression, and catabolism syndrome. Nutr Clin Pract. 2017;32:121S–7S.
2. Herndon DN, Tompkins RG. Support of the metabolic response to burn injury. Lancet. 2004;363:1895–902.
3. Hazeldine J, Hampson P, Lord JM. The diagnostic and prognostic value of systems biology research in major traumatic and thermal injury: a review. Burns Trauma. 2016;4:33.

4. Porter C, Tompkins RG, Finnerty CC, Sidossis LS, Suman OE, Herndon DN. The metabolic stress response to burn trauma: current understanding and therapies. Lancet. 2016;388:1417–26.

5. Rousseau AF, Losser MR, Ichai C, Berger MM. ESPEN endorsed recommendations: nutritional therapy in major burns. Clin Nutr. 2013;32:497–502.

6. Jafari P, Thomas A, Haselbach D, Watfa W, Pantet O, Michetti M, Raffoul W, Applegate LA, Augsburger M, Berger MM. Trace element intakes should be revisited in burn nutrition protocols: A cohort study. Clin Nutr. 2017;pii:S0261–5614(17)30119-X. doi:10.1016/j.clnu.2017.03.028. [Epub ahead of print] PMID: 28455105.

7. Jeschke MG, Gauglitz GG, Kulp GA, Finnerty CC, Williams FN, Kraft R, Suman OE, Mlcak RP, Herndon DN. Long-term persistence of the pathophysiologic response to severe burn injury. PLoS One. 2011;6:e21245.

8. Stanojcic M, Finnerty CC, Jeschke MG. Anabolic and anticatabolic agents in critical care. Curr Opin Crit Care. 2016;22:325–31.

9. Williams FN, Branski LK, Jeschke MG, Herndon DN. What, how, and how much should patients with burns be fed? Surg Clin North Am. 2011;91:609–29.

10. Patterson BW, Nguyen T, Pierre E, Herndon DN, Wolfe RR. Urea and protein metabolism in burned children: effect of dietary protein intake. Metabolism. 1997;46:573–8.

11. Pantet O, Stoecklin P, Vernay A, Berger MM. Impact of decreasing energy intakes in major burn patients: a 15 year retrospective cohort study. Clin Nutr. 2017;36:818–24.

12. Lin JJ, Chung XJ, Yang CY, Lau HL. A meta-analysis of trials using the intention to treat principle for glutamine supplementation in critically ill patients with burn. Burns. 2013;39:565–70.

13. Burke JF, Wolfe RR, Mullany CJ, Mathews DE, Bier DM. Glucose requirements following burn injury. Parameters of optimal glucose infusion and possible hepatic and respiratory abnormalities following excessive glucose intake. Ann Surg. 1979;190:274–85.

14. Stoecklin P, Delodder F, Pantet O, Berger MM. Moderate glycemic control safe in critically ill adult burn patients—a 15 year cohort study. Burns. 2016;42:63–70.

15. Kahn SA, Beers RJ, Lentz CW. Resuscitation after severe burn injury using high-dose ascorbic acid: a retrospective review. J Burn Care Res. 2011;32:110–7.

16. Rousseau AF, Damas P, Ledoux D, Cavalier E. Effect of cholecalciferol recommended daily allowances on vitamin D status and fibroblast growth factor-23: an observational study in acute burn patients. Burns. 2014;40:865–70.

17. Klein GL, Herndon DN, Chen TC, Kulp G, Holick MF. Standard multivitamin supplementation does not improve vitamin D insufficiency after burns. J Bone Miner Metab. 2009;27:502–6.
18. Ebid AA, El-Shamy SM, Amer MA. Effect of vitamin D supplementation and isokinetic training on muscle strength, explosive strength, lean body mass and gait in severely burned children: a randomized controlled trial. Burns. 2017;43:357–65.
19. Reeves PT, Herndon DN, Tanksley JD, Jennings K, Klein GL, Mlcak RP, Clayton RP, Crites NN, Hays JP, Andersen C, Lee JO, Meyer W, Suman OE, Finnerty CC. Five-year outcomes after long-term Oxandrolone administration in severely burned children: a randomized clinical trial. Shock. 2016;45:367–74.
20. Li H, Guo Y, Yang Z, Roy M, Guo Q. The efficacy and safety of oxandrolone treatment for patients with severe burns: a systematic review and meta-analysis. Burns. 2016;42:717–27.
21. Sudenis T, Hall K, Cartotto R. Enteral nutrition: what the dietitian prescribes is not what the burn patient gets! J Burn Care Res. 2015;36:297–305.
22. Berger MM, Shenkin A. Trace element requirements in critically ill burned patients. J Trace Elem Med Biol. 2007;21(Suppl 1):44–8.
23. Sakallioglu AE, Basaran O, Karakayali H, Ozdemir BH, Yucel M, Arat Z, Haberal M. Interactions of systemic immune response and local wound healing in different burn depths: an experimental study on rats. J Burn Care Res. 2006;27:357–66.
24. Farina JA Jr, Rosique MJ, Rosique RG. Curbing inflammation in burn patients. Int J Inflam. 2013;2013:715645.

Chapter 7
Obesity

David C. Frankenfield

7.1   Introduction

Obesity is a form of malnutrition in which an imbalance between energy intake and expenditure leads to accumulation of body fat, which in turn can alter body function and increase mortality risk. Obesity is defined, simply, as excess body fat. This may be the only simple aspect of the condition. The rest is fraught with uncertainty, starting with the body fat threshold to define the condition. Typically, the stated thresholds are 25% of body weight in men and 35% in women [1], but there is no criterion standard for defining excess body fat. Furthermore, there are several obesity phenotypes [2], the morbidity and mortality risks can be different by phenotype [3], and the phenotypes can be difficult to identify [2]. There is a possibility in critical care that obesity may be protective to some degree (the obesity paradox) [4]. Many nutrition care practices for the critically ill obese patient are adopted from evidence-based recommendations made for nonobese patients [5, 6]. It is telling that among the eight questions

D.C. Frankenfield, MS, RD
Department of Clinical Nutrition, Department of Nursing,
Penn State Health System, Milton S. Hershey Medical Center,
Pennsylvania, USA
e-mail: dfrankenfield@pennstatehealth.psu.edu

© Springer International Publishing AG 2018   89
M.M. Berger (ed.), *Critical Care Nutrition Therapy
for Non-nutritionists*, https://doi.org/10.1007/978-3-319-58652-6_7

posed for nutrition care of the obese critically ill patient in the ASPEN/SCCM guideline, all are answered by expert consensus (the lowest category of evidence) [5].

7.2   Specific Metabolic and Nutritional Characteristics

The primary characteristic of obesity is excess body fat. Accompanying this excess in body fat are disturbances in fat-free mass, either an increase or a decrease [2]. An obese person with low fat-free mass is often said to have sarcopenic obesity. The other group might be said to have hypertrophic obesity due to an increase in muscle mass presumably the result of carrying the excess body fat. These two categories exist on a continuum, so there are innumerable combinations of fat mass and fat-free mass possible among obese people.

Though obesity is excess body fat, it is most often described and diagnosed with body mass index (BMI, kg/ht^2) because height and weight measurements are easier to obtain than measurements of body composition. However, BMI is a measure of mass and not composition, so it does not accurately categorize all patients into obese or nonobese groups. BMI of 30 kg/m^2 is considered the threshold for obesity and so in theory should equate to body fat 25% in men and 35% in women. The actual threshold body fat percentages for BMI 30 however are closer to 30% in men and 45% in women [7]. Furthermore, BMI sensitivity for identifying obesity is low (about 43%) [8], and specificity is unclear (the index had 96% specificity in one study but misclassified 32% of men and 17% of women as obese in another study) [8, 9].

As defined by BMI ≥ 30.0 kg/m^2, fasting obese critically ill patients typically have insulin resistance and are more likely to be hyperglycemic [10, 11]. Despite a similar muscle breakdown rate (0.4% per of muscle mass per day), obese patients direct a smaller percentage of the resulting amino acids back toward protein synthesis (58 vs. 66%) and lose a higher portion of nitrogen in their urine [11]. There is a greater reliance on protein and carbohydrate as fuel sources despite the large depot of fat contained in adipose tissue [11]. This is in direct contrast to healthy people in whom an increasing body fat is associated with protein-sparing during a fast [2].

7.3   Timing of Nutritional Intervention

Nutrition support for critically ill obese people should be initiated within the same time frame as for nonobese patients. There should be no assumption that obese patients have adequate energy stores and therefore can weather critical illness more successfully without nutrient intake. Many obese patients suffer from sarcopenia that may go unrecognized because of their body habitus. Furthermore, metabolic alterations are common in the obese that accelerate the catabolism of body protein. Ironically then, despite a surfeit of stored energy, the obese person may reach a critical level of protein depletion before a nonobese person. Enteral nutrition should therefore be initiated within 24–48 h of admission to the critical care unit [5].

7.4   Feeding Route

As with nonobese patients, the critically ill obese patient should be fed via the enteral route whenever possible. Of note, it is important to ascertain if the patient has had bariatric surgery resulting in altered gastric or small intestinal anatomy as this may in turn alter the choice for tube location (distal to the gastric pouch), feeding infusion method or feeding type (peptide rather than polymeric if there has been significant small intestine exclusion). Although most critically ill patients independent of their obesity status are fed by continuous infusion, in the case of bariatric surgery patients, there is no alternative but to infuse the feeding continuously.

7.5   Specific Needs of the Category

As stated above, the timing and route of nutrition support of the obese critically ill patient is the same as for nonobese patients. The major difference between these groups in terms of nutrition care plan is the uncertainty in the determination of metabolic demand and in the amount of this demand that should be fed.

Description of the nutritional needs of the obese critically ill patient is complicated by the choice of how to index the requirement. In absolute terms, the obese person will typically have higher energy expenditure and protein breakdown than a nonobese person, owing to the larger body mass and the correlation between body weight and fat-free mass. A meaningful comparison between obese and nonobese must therefore be indexed to a parameter of body size. Depending on the index, the differences in energy and protein demand between obese and nonobese individuals become less obvious, or they may even become reversed (Table 7.1). Furthermore, care must be taken in how metabolic requirements are indexed because the index itself can be erroneous.

TABLE 7.1 Feeding strategy according to types of obese patients

Requirements	Healthy and sarcopenic obese	Obese post-bypass surgery
Location of EN feeding tube extremity	Gastric or post-pyloric based on gastric function and aspiration risk	Distal to the gastric pouch
Types of EN feeds	Polymeric	Polymeric or possibly semi-elemental depending on the degree of intestinal exclusion
Micronutrients	Standard	Supplements due to malabsorption

7.5.1 Energy

The sum total of macronutrient utilization in the human body is reflected in the daily energy expenditure. Total energy expenditure can be partitioned into resting energy expenditure (REE), expenditure associated with digestion and metabolism of food, and expenditure due to physical activity. In the critically ill patient, REE is elevated to varying degrees by the inflammatory response. The thermogenic effect of feeding is often assumed to increase energy expenditure by about 10%, but the effect is minimized or possibly nonexistent in many critical care patients by virtue of the continuous feeding state methods most often used in this population. Energy expended in physical activity can be highly variable and difficult to quantify, being influenced by the degree of agitation or sedation and the frequency and duration of routine care practices (e.g., bathing, dressing changes). Although individual activities can transiently increase expenditure by 30% or more, the overall effect in 24 h is on the order of 5–10%. These features of total daily energy expenditure do not differ between obese and nonobese patients.

Table 7.2 is a compilation of REE variables from metabolic studies in obese and nonobese critically ill, mechanically ventilated patients [12, 13]. As can be seen in the table, both groups have a high incidence of hypermetabolism. However, although body weight (BW) is 53% higher in the obese than the nonobese patients, the resting metabolic rate is increased by only 22%, implying a lower severity of hypermetabolism compared to nonobese patients. There is no ratio index that normalizes the difference in REE between these two groups. Indexing to body weight creates the appearance of a low REE in the obese group. Indexing to either metabolically active body weight or ideal body weight creates the appearance of a high REE in the obese relative to the nonobese group, implying that obese patients have a higher degree of hypermetabolism. However, all of these ratio indices assume a zero-intercept (i.e., REE = 0 + A(wt)), but in fact they all have intercepts that do not equal zero. Ignoring this fact

TABLE 7.2 REE data in obese and nonobese patients showing variations depending on method of indexing

Variable	Obese (*n* = 105)	Nonobese (*n* = 104)	*p*-Value
Body weight (BW) (kg)	117 ± 38	73 ± 12	0.000
Body mass index (kg/m^2)	40.0 ± 12.2	25.0 ± 2.9	0.000
REE (kcal/day)	2222 ± 573	1811 ± 410	0.000
REE (kcal/kg BW)	19.6 ± 4.5	25.0 ± 4.1	0.000
REE (kcal/kg adjusted BW)	27.9 ± 4.6	25.0 ± 4.1	0.000
REE (kcal/kg ideal BW)	33.6 ± 5.9	27.7 ± 4.5	0.000
REE (regression with BW)	2006 ± 476	2028 ± 473	0.758
Hypermetabolism (percent incidence[*])	71	78	0.291

[*]Percentage of patients with REE >10% above estimated healthy REE

creates error in the estimate of REE from body weight. Indexing RMR to body weight by using a regression method shows that the values equalize between the obese and non-obese groups. Ignoring the *y*-intercept therefore seems to be a major reason why ratio methods of predicting REE fail, and this is why such methods should not be employed. Proper indexing by regression, holding body size as a covariate, shows that REE is not different between obese and nonobese patients.

Measurement with indirect calorimetry is the gold standard method of determining REE, but the procedure must be repeated every 3–4 days to remain accurate because REE is not constant in the critically ill [14]. Indirect calorimetry is expensive and labor intensive, and many patients cannot be measured (e.g., patients with high FIO$_2$, air leaks, or unsteady respiratory parameters). Predictive equations are therefore the most common method for determining REE in critically ill patients [15]. As above, any prediction method that utilizes a ratio of energy to body mass is likely to fail because ratio methods ignore non-zero intercepts in the relation between the energy and mass variables. The Penn State equations seem to be the most reliable of the Eqs. 12–14. They are regression equations rather than ratios. They capture day-to-day variability in REE by using body temperature and minute ventilation, and they capture the effect of body mass by using the Mifflin St. Jeor equation (REE (kcal/day) = Wt(10) + Ht(6.25) − Age (5) + Male(166) − 161). Compiling all validation data from the authors of the equation, the accuracy rate is 72% in nonobese patients and 70% in obese patients up to a BMI of 80 kg/m^2. In two subjects with BMI >100, the equation failed (overestimating the measured metabolic rate in both) [12–14].

7.5.2   Protein

Protein requirements in the critically ill are a function of fat-free mass and degree of catabolism. Determination of protein requirements is most often weight based, relying on associations between body weight and fat-free mass. In the obese patient, weight-based estimates of protein requirement will be compromised by the fact that the relation between weight and fat-free mass is altered. Validated prediction equations for protein requirement do not exist. Fortunately, measurement of protein requirement by nitrogen balance is a much less involved process than is indirect calorimetry for measurement of energy demand, and so it is more accessible, but it does require adequate renal function and accurate urine collection.

Independent of the exact body demand for energy and protein, controversy exists as to the optimal intake of each [3, 5, 6, 15]. Alberda et al. [3] observed that increasing the energy and protein intake in critically ill patients was associated with a decrease in mortality in patients with BMI <25 kg/m^2 and >35 kg/m^2 but not in patients with BMI between 25 and 34.9 kg/m^2. These thresholds do not correspond with the traditional thresholds for underweight or obesity, and this may be an illustration of the fact that BMI is an index of mass and not composition. One interpretation of the Alberda et al. result is that patients who most benefit from increasing the intake of energy and protein are those with reduced muscle mass as one would expect to encounter such patients in the highest and lowest BMI categories.

7.6   Monitoring of the Intervention

Biochemical monitoring of the obese patient should be the same as for nonobese patients. Measurement of nitrogen loss in the urine may be more important in the obese than the nonobese patient because the typical method of calculation of protein requirement is based on body weight and this may be disrupted by the change in body weight and composition typical of obese patients.

Gastrointestinal tolerance to enteral feeding should be monitored. The method is not different between the obese and nonobese patient, but particular to the obese patient, abdominal distention may be more difficult to appreciate due to body habitus.

7.7   Conclusion

Nutrition care of the obese patient in the critical care unit is the same for the most part as the nutrition care of their non-obese counterparts. Early initiation of therapy by the enteral route is the standard of care. Blood glucose should be controlled to <180 mg/dL (<10 mmol/L). Less certain is the determination of how much energy and protein is demanded by the obese body and how much of that demand should be fed.

There is broad consensus that protein intake should not be limited, but there is uncertainty as to what the protein requirement is. Contrarily, there is no consensus as to the percentage of energy demand that should be fed to the critically ill obese patient, especially early in their critical care course.

Equations exist for the calculation of energy and protein needs, but equation reliability is reduced, especially at BMI above 80 kg/m². Particularly for protein but also possibly for energy, measurement of the need may be more important for the obese patient than the nonobese in order to avoid the higher risk of error in the obese patient.

References

1. AACE/ACE Obesity Task Force. AACE/ACE position statement on the prevention, diagnosis, and treatment of obesity. Endocr Pract. 1998;4:297–350.
2. Dulloo AG, Solinas JJ, Montani JP, Schultz Y. Body composition phenotypes in pathways to obesity and the metabolic syndrome. Int J Obes. 2010;34:S4–S17.
3. Alberda C, Gramlich L, Jones N, Jeejeebhoy K, Day AG, Dhaliwal R, Heyland DK. The relationship between nutritional intake and clinical outcomes in critically ill patients: results of an international multicenter observational study. Intensive Care Med. 2009;35:1728–37.
4. Akinnusi ME, Pineda LA, Solh AA. Effect of obesity on intensive care morbidity and mortality: a meta analysis. Crit Care Med. 2008;36:151–8.
5. McClave SA, Taylor BE, Martindale RG, et al. Guidelines for the provision and assessment of nutrition support therapy in the adult critically ill patient: society of critical care medicine (SCCM) and American society for parenteral and enteral nutrition (ASPEN). J Parenter Enter Nutr. 2016;40:159–211.
6. Preiser JC, van Zanten ARH, Merger MM, et al. Metabolic and nutritional support of critically ill patients: consensus and controversies. Crit Care. 2015;19:1–11.
7. Pasco JA, Holloway KL, Dobbins AG, Kotowicz MA, Williams LJ, Brennan SL. Body mass index and measures of body fat for defining obesity and underweight: a cross-sectional population-based study. BMC Obes. 2014;1:9. doi:10.1186/2052-9538-1-9.
8. Romero-Corral A, Somers VK, Sierra-Johnson J, Thomas RJ, Bailey KR, Collazo-Clavell ML, Allison TG, Korinek J, Batsis JA, Lopez-Jimenez F. Accuracy of body mass index to diagnose obesity in the US adult population. Int J Obes. 2008;32: 959–66.

9. Gallagher D, Heymsfield SB, Heo M, Jebb SA, Murgatroyd PR, Sakamoto Y. Healthy percentage body fat ranges: an approach for developing guidelines based on body mass index. Am J Clin Nutr. 2000;72:694–701.

10. Gallagher D, DeLegge M. Body composition (sarcopenia) in obese patients: implications for care in the intensive care unit. J Parenter Enter Nutr. 2011;35(5 Suppl):21S–8S.

11. Jeevanandam M, Young DH, Schiller WR. Obesity and the metabolic response to severe multiple trauma in man. J Clin Invest. 1991;87:262–9.

12. Frankenfield DC, Schubert A, Alam S, Cooney RN. Validation study of predictive equations for resting metabolic rate in critically ill patients. J Parenter Enter Nutr. 2009;33:27–36.

13. Frankenfield DC, Ashcraft CM, Galvan DA. Prediction of resting metabolic rate in critically ill patients at the extremes of body mass index. J Parenter Enter Nutr. 2013;37:361–7.

14. Frankenfield DC, Ashcraft CM, Galvan DA. Longitudinal prediction of metabolic rate in critically ill patients. J Parenter Enter Nutr. 2012;36:700–12.

15. Heyland DK, Cahill N, Day AG. Optimal amount of calories for critically ill patients: depends on how you slice the cake. Crit Care Med. 2011;39:2619–26.

Chapter 8
Acute Kidney Injury With and Without Renal Replacement Therapy

Antoine Schneider

8.1 Introduction

Acute kidney injury (AKI) is common and severe in critically ill patients [1]. AKI is associated with alteration in protein, glucid and lipid metabolism as well as pro-inflammatory actions and alteration of antioxidant systems. These changes concur in an increased catabolism leading to lean mass and fat wasting. The occurrence of AKI in critically ill patients is particularly devastating in terms of nutritional status since those patients are already at risk of nutritional deficiency because of prolonged hospital stay, limited mobilization, inflammatory state, sickness-associated anorexia as well as potential delay in nutritional support initiation. Altogether, the combination of AKI and critical illness frequently leads to protein-energy wasting (PEW), a syndrome with prognostic implications, particularly when renal replacement therapy (RRT) is required [2]. Therefore, early and focused nutritional support must be provided in critically ill patients with AKI.

A. Schneider
Service de Médecine Intensive Adulte et Centre de Brûlés,
Centre Hospitalier et Universitaire Vaudois (CHUV),
Avenue du Bugnon 46, 1011 Lausanne, Switzerland
e-mail: antoine.schneider@chuv.ch

© Springer International Publishing AG 2018   99
M.M. Berger (ed.), *Critical Care Nutrition Therapy*
for Non-nutritionists, https://doi.org/10.1007/978-3-319-58652-6_8

This chapter reviews specific metabolic and nutritional characteristics of critically ill patients with AKI and presents the basics of appropriate nutritional support.

8.2   Metabolic and Nutritional Characteristics of Patients with AKI

AKI profoundly modifies metabolic and nutritional characteristics of the patients. It is associated with alterations of protein, glucid and lipid metabolism and increased pro-oxidant state. When RRT needs to be applied, further alterations are observed secondary to loss of nutrients through the effluent and substrate delivery through dialysate or substitution solutions.

8.2.1   AKI Metabolic and Nutritional Implications

8.2.1.1   Protein Metabolism

AKI is associated with increased protein catabolism. In addition to inflammation and stress, common to all critically ill patients, AKI-associated protein catabolism seems to be mediated by metabolic acidosis through facilitated branched amino acids (leucin, isoleucine, valin) degradation [3] and activation of ATP-ubiquitin-dependant proteolytic system [4]. Metabolic acidosis also increases cortisol secretion, which further aggravates this phenomenon. The resulting protein deficit can further be enhanced when a low-protein diet is prescribed to try and avoid RRT.

8.2.1.2   Glucose Metabolism

AKI is characterized by hyperglycaemia due to peripheral insulin resistance [4] and accelerated hepatic neoglucogenesis [5]. This aggravates stress hyperglycaemia, commonly observed in critically ill patients. Hyperglycaemia is potentially harmful as suggested by observational data showing a strong association between elevated blood sugar levels and adverse events in hospitalized patients. Glucose intolerance is particularly common during RRT perhaps due to a loss of chrome in the effluent [6]. Indeed, chrome is involved in glucose control through chromodulin, a molecule, which binds to activated insulin receptor and stimulates its kinase activity. In rare instances, impaired renal neoglucogenesis might lead to a tendency to *hypoglycaemia*.

8.2.1.3   Inflammatory State

Inflammatory state is a hallmark of AKI. It might be part of the pathological process leading to AKI, but recent data suggest that AKI itself stimulates pro-inflammatory cytokines release, which affects the immune system and organ function [7, 8]. This enhanced inflammatory state further aggravates catabolism, induces anorexia and might be associated with further deterioration of patients' nutritional status.

8.2.2   RRT-Associated Thermal Losses

RRT is associated with important thermal losses linked to the extra-corporeal circuit. In a recent study, hypothermia (<35 °C) was observed in 44% of patients [9]. In fully sedated paralysed patients, those thermic losses might be of benefit as they decrease baseline metabolic demand and therefore VO_2. In all other cases, the body's reaction to normalize temperature (chills) will lead to increased metabolic needs.

8.2.3   RRT-Associated Nutrient Losses

The amount of nutrient loss through the effluent depends on many factors: type of filter (permeability coefficient and surface), RRT dose and modality.

Table 8.1 Summary recommendations for nutritional management in AKI

• Recognize PEW and start nutritional support early
• Reference weight for calculation should be based on anamnestic value rather than measured weight (fluid overload)
• Introduce enteral feeding within 24–48 h if possible
• Aim to achieve a total energy intake of 20–30 kcal/kg/day
• Account for nutrient loss and intake through RRT
• Restrict potassium phosphate and fluid administration
• Target blood glucose values between 110 and 150 mg/dL (6.1–8.3 mmol/L)
• Use calorimetry if available

8.2.3.1   Proteins and Amino Acids

RRT is associated with amino acid loss (approximately 0.2 g/L of effluent). According to the technique used, this loss can reach 25 g/day (Table 8.1). In CVVHDF mode, amino acid clearance ranges from 0 (aspartate) to 45.5 mL/min (tyrosine) [10].

8.2.3.2   Glucids

Glucose is a small molecule, which is very easily be removed by RRT. Without adequate substitution, RRT would lead to massive glucose loss (up to 60 g/day) and hypoglycaemia. In order to compensate for or minimize those losses, substitution fluids and dialysis solutions contain glucose. In CVVH (or CVVHDF) mode, solutions with more than 1% glucose lead to a net glucose intake. Dialysis solutions used in CVVHD mode typically have a glucose concentration corresponding to the physiological blood glucose level (1 g/L).

8.2.3.3   Lipids

Most lipids in the plasma circulate in the form of lipoproteins (chylomicrons, VLDL, LDL or HDL). These molecules are large and their removal by RRT is minimal. Only short or middle-size chain fatty acids would be susceptible to cross membrane pores; however, such molecules are 95% albumin bound, and their losses are therefore also minimal.

8.2.3.4   Micronutrients

In critically ill patients with AKI low blood levels of selenium, β-carotene and vitamin C were repeatedly observed [6]. This deficit is particularly severe during RRT since significant amount of vitamin C, selenium, chrome, zinc, thiamine and copper are removed in the effluent [6, 11]. Zinc plasma levels are usually maintained since substitution solutions contain this element. Loss of micronutrients in particular selenium, zinc, β-carotene and vitamin C is thought to be associated with increased oxidative stress through alterations of glutathione peroxidases (GPX), which correspond to the first line of antioxidant defence of the organism.

8.2.4   RRT-Associated Energy and Substrate Delivery

Beyond potential glucose delivery already mentioned, some components of the RRT solutions might represent a substrate source.

8.2.4.1   Citrate

Citrate ($C_6H_5O_7$) is increasingly used for regional anticoagulation of RRT circuit. Citrate can directly be used at the mitochondrial level and generates 3 kcal/g (0.59 kcal/mmol) [12]. With standard regimen, calorie intake associated with citrate can be over 250 kcal/day. Of note, calculation of citrate-associated energy delivery should account for citrate removal at the filter level. In CVVHD mode, close to 50% of administered citrate is removed through the dialysate. The amount of citrate delivered to the patient is influenced by set blood flow (the higher blood flow the more citrate needs to be administered) and the RRT dose (the higher the dose, the higher the removal).

8.2.4.2   Lactate

Lactate, a precursor of renal neoglucogenesis, has long represented a buffer in substitution solutions. Its utilization is now largely decreasing due to the popularity of bicarbonate-based solutions. Lactate corresponds to an energy source, generating approximately 60 kJ/h (345 kcal/day).

8.3   Timing of Nutritional Intervention

There is no specific data on the timing of nutritional support introduction in AKI. Similar to any critically ill patient, introducing enteral feeding within 24–48 h of admission seems appropriate [13].

8.4   Specific Nutritional Needs of Patients with AKI

8.4.1   Energy Intake

Energy requirements appear to be mostly dependent on underlying disease, baseline nutritional status rather than renal disease itself [14]. However, as already mentioned, AKI identifies a population at risk of PEW, and the introduction of an early and adequate nutritional support must represent a priority in such patients.

The European and American nutrition society as well as the KDIGO (Kidney Disease—Improving Global Outcomes) society recommend to achieve a total energy intake of 20–30 kcal/kg/day in patients with any stage of AKI [5, 14, 15]. This amount might be increased to 35 kcal/kg/h during RRT [5]. In obese or largely malnourished patients, specific adjustments are necessary [16]. As previously mentioned, the amount of energy provided by RRT solutions must be integrated in the caloric intake of the patient.

8.4.2 Choice of Solutions and Substrate

8.4.2.1 AKI Without RRT

In the context of AKI, potassium, phosphate and fluid intake should be restricted. In enterally fed patients, this translates into the use of high-energy (concentrated) solutions to minimize fluid intake.

As for most ICU patients, glucids should represent the dominant energy source for AKI patients without exceeding 60% of total energy intake to prevent de novo hepatic lipogenesis (Table 8.2).

Lipids should not represent more than 20–30% of total energy delivery. There is currently no data enabling the recommendation of a particular fatty acid composition.

Daily protein intake is more subject to discussion. When BUN >20 mmol/L, most clinicians would decrease the protein intake to <1 g/kg/day to minimize urea generation. However, there is little evidence that this practice actually prevents further kidney injury or delay RRT. The KDIGO society recommends *against* this practice [5]. Current recommendations are to administer 0.8–1 g/kg/day of proteins in non-catabolic patients without need for dialysis, 1.0–1.5 g/kg/day in patients on RRT and up to a maximum of 1.7 g/kg/day in patients on continuous RRT [5, 14].

TABLE 8.2 Recommended energy and substrate targets

	Recommended daily intake	
Substrate	No RRT	RRT
Total energy	20–35 kcal/kg according to sedation level	
Glucids	4–5 g/kg/day	
Proteins	1 g/kg	1.7 → 2.0–2.5 g/kg
Lipids	20–25% of total energy	

8.4.3   Micronutrients and Antioxidants

Since blood concentrations of selenium, copper and other micronutrients are low in AKI particularly when RRT is provided, supplementation could be necessary. The evidence supporting this practice remains however limited. Currently, commercially available micronutrient preparations are dedicated to total parenteral nutrition and not specifically adapted to AKI. Some experts recommend prescribing micronutrients to patients with RRT for AKI even when enteral nutrition is provided. A dose corresponding to twice that administered for total parenteral nutrition is commonly advocated. Experts also commonly recommend the prescription of 100 µg of selenium and 100 mg of thiamine. The supporting evidence for this practice remains low in the current literature.

Vitamin C substitution during AKI is debated. It could worsen AKI by favouring the formation of oxalate crystals. However, as already mentioned, patients with AKI often have low blood levels of vitamin C, in particular when receiving RRT. Since low vitamin C levels are associated with increased rate of cardiovascular complications and mortality, a supplementation might be considered.

Of note, the fact that a substance is removed by RRT does not automatically imply that its substitution would be beneficial or indicated. Indeed, the amount of this removal must be weighed against the systemic turnover of the molecule. The substitution route also matters. For instance, during parenteral nutrition, amino acid losses through the effluent are higher than during enteral nutrition. Indeed, losses are proportional to plasma concentration, and it seems like 10% of infused amino acids are directly lost [4].

8.4.4   Glycaemic Control

As presented above, AKI is associated with insulin resistance and decreased neoglucogenesis. Exogenous insulin however remains efficient and is very frequently necessary. Insulin therapy targeting blood glucose values between 110 and 150 mg/dL (6.1–8.3 mmol/L) is recommended by the KDIGO society [5].

8.5   Feeding Route

Enteral route should be favoured as much as possible in patients with AKI [5]. Despite theoretical concerns regarding uraemia-associated gut motility limitations, enteral nutrition is usually effective and well tolerated. However, full administration of energetic requirement remains can be difficult and combination of enteral and parenteral route or rarely total parenteral nutrition might be required.

8.6   Monitoring

Formal evaluation of nutritional status is particularly difficult in AKI. Indeed, common evaluation tools are altered both by critical illness and renal failure [8]. Typically, fluid overload makes weight estimation difficult. Reference weight for calculation must rely on patient history (usual body weight) or on ideal weight rather than actual measurements. Similarly, fluid accumulation in subcutaneous tissues alters anthropometric measurements such as "skin fold" and muscle volume. Protein blood levels (particularly albumin particular) are largely altered by volume status and systemic inflammation. Nitrogen balance is very imprecise in AKI but can be used in patients on RRT (effluent needs to be analysed) to determine catabolic state and protein needs. Its utilization remains however limited in clinical practice. The gold standard for nutritional evaluation in critical care and in AKI in particular remains indirect calorimetry. Unfortunately, this technique has low availability and is associated with technical limitations (low precision if FIO_2 >60%, gas leaks etc.).

Practically, all these elements need to be integrated taking into account their limitations as well as clinical context to evaluate patient's nutritional status and establish a personalized nutritional plan. Daily and cumulated caloric balance are a pragmatic way to move forward.

8.7   Conclusion

Patients with AKI are at high risk of PEW through accelerated catabolism, low nutritional intake and additional losses through RRT when administered. The early introduction of nutritional support should be a therapeutic priority in those patients. This support should aim at delivering relatively high quantity of energy and proteins and substitute hydrosoluble elements.

Conflict of Interests   The author declares he has no conflict of interest relative to this book chapter.

References

1. Hoste EA, Bagshaw SM, Bellomo R, et al. Epidemiology of acute kidney injury in critically ill patients: the multinational AKI-EPI study. Intensive Care Med. 2015;41(8):1411–23.
2. Fiaccadori E, Lombardi M, Leonardi S, Rotelli CF, Tortorella G, Borghetti A. Prevalence and clinical outcome associated with preexisting malnutrition in acute renal failure: a prospective cohort study. J Am Soc Nephrol. 1999;10(3):581–93.
3. Wooley JA, Btaiche IF, Good KL. Metabolic and nutritional aspects of acute renal failure in critically ill patients requiring continuous renal replacement therapy. Nutr Clin Pract. 2005;20(2):176–91.
4. Leverve XM, Cano NJ. Nutritional management in acute illness and acute kidney insufficiency. Contrib Nephrol. 2007;156:112–8.
5. KDIGO. KDIGO clinical practice guideline for acute kidney injury. Kidney Int. 2012;2(1).
6. Story D, Ronco C, Bellomo R. Trace element and vitamin concentrations and losses in critically ill patients treated with continuous venovenous hemofiltration. Crit Care Med. 1999;27:220–3.

 7. Faubel S, Edelstein CL. Mechanisms and mediators of lung injury after acute kidney injury. Nat Rev Nephrol. 2016;12(1):48–60.

 8. Fiaccadori E, Regolisti G, Maggiore U. Specialized nutritional support interventions in critically ill patients on renal replacement therapy. Curr Opin Clin Nutr Metab Care. 2013;16(2):217–24.

 9. Akhoundi A, Singh B, Vela M, et al. Incidence of adverse events during continuous renal replacement therapy. Blood Purif. 2015;39(4):333–9.

10. Bellomo R, Tan HK, Bhonagiri S, et al. High protein intake during continuous hemodiafiltration: impact on amino acids and nitrogen balance. Int J Artif Organs. 2002;25(4):261–8.

11. Ben-Hamouda N, Charriere M, Voirol P, Berger MM. Massive copper and selenium losses cause life-threatening deficiencies during prolonged continuous renal replacement. Nutrition. 2017;34:71–5.

12. Oudemans-van Straaten HM, Kellum JA, Bellomo R. Clinical review: anticoagulation for continuous renal replacement therapy—heparin or citrate? Crit Care. 2011;15(1):202.

13. Reintam Blaser A, Starkopf J, Alhazzani W, et al. Early enteral nutrition in critically ill patients: ESICM clinical practice guidelines. Intensive Care Med. 2017;43(3):380–98.

14. Cano NJ, Aparicio M, Brunori G, et al. ESPEN guidelines on parenteral nutrition: adult renal failure. Clin Nutr. 2009;28(4):401–14.

15. Brown RO, Compher C, American society for Parental, Enteral Nutrition Board of Directors. A.S.P.E.N. Clinical guidelines: nutrition support in adult acute and chronic renal failure. JPEN J Parenter Enteral Nutr. 2010;34(4):366–77.

16. Cano N, Fiaccadori E, Tesinsky P, et al. ESPEN guidelines on enteral nutrition: adult renal failure. Clin Nutr. 2006;25(2):295–310.

Chapter 9
Enteral Feeding and Noninvasive Ventilation

Jean-Michel Constantin, Lionel Bouvet, and Sébastien Perbet

9.1 Introduction

In the last decades, noninvasive ventilation (NIV) has been increasingly applied in a growing number of acute care settings and conditions for prevention or treatment of acute respiratory failure (ARF). Its efficacy has been evaluated in several randomized trials, and it is currently considered a first-line treatment in some common conditions such as chronic obstructive pulmonary disease (COPD) exacerbation, cardiogenic pulmonary edema, pneumonia in immunosuppressed patients, and postoperative ARF [1]. However, so far its benefit on survival has not yet been demonstrated for many indications, and its utilization is more and more challenging at least for ARF; physicians' daily use of NIV in acute care setting and the question of nutritional support for

J.-M. Constantin (✉) • S. Perbet
Department of Perioperative Medicine,
University Hospital of Clermont-Ferrand,
Clermont-Ferrand, France
e-mail: jmconstantin@chu-clermontferrand.fr

L. Bouvet
Department of Anesthesia and Intensive Care,
Hospice Civils Lyon, Lyon, France

© Springer International Publishing AG 2018 111
M.M. Berger (ed.), *Critical Care Nutrition Therapy for Non-nutritionists*, https://doi.org/10.1007/978-3-319-58652-6_9

patients on NIV remain a hot topic. Early enteral nutrition (EN) is recommended for mechanically ventilated patients in several studies and guidelines [2]. Enteral nutrition reportedly reduces the duration of mechanical ventilation and hospitalization and enhances patient survival. However, the effects of early EN on NIV have not been investigated extensively. In addition, EN has shown adverse effects, including critical ones. Patients receiving NIV may experience various complications, including airway problems (vomiting, increased sputum, mucus plugging, and atelectasis) and other problems (discomfort, pneumothorax, hypotension, cardiac rhythm disturbances, and anxiety). Enteral nutrition may worsen these complications, especially airway complications, possibly leading to critical problems, such as pneumonia and airway obstruction. Moreover, unlike for invasive ventilation, no methods of airway protection have been established for NIV. Despite the advantages of EN in patients with acute respiratory failure, the effects of EN in patients receiving NIV have not been clarified. Only one study directly related to this topic has been published [3]. In this monocentric retrospective study, the authors analyzed 107 patients over 8 years admitted in their ICU for ARF treated by NIV, 60 with EN and 47 without. The rate of airway complications was significantly higher (53% vs. 32%, $P = 0.03$), and the median NIV duration was significantly longer (16 vs. 8 days, $P = 0.02$) in subjects who received EN than in those who did not. No difference in hospital or overall mortality was shown. They concluded that among subjects receiving NIV, EN was associated with increased risk of airway complications but did not affect mortality. Because no conclusion could be drawn from this study, and in the absence of ongoing RCT, a physiological approach must be proposed for daily practice in ICU setting.

9.2   Noninvasive Ventilation

In critically ill patients, after surgery or due to nonsurgical diseases, respiratory function may be substantially modified independently of initial lung injury. Anesthesia, postoperative pain and surgery, particularly when the site of the surgery approaches the diaphragm, bed rest, inflammation and fluid overload often induce respiratory modifications such as hypoxemia, atelectasis, and diaphragm dysfunction. Moreover, swallowing disorders and vomiting may cause aspiration. These disorders will also impact on the oral feeding capacity of the patients, as well as on EN tolerance.

9.3   Technical Considerations About NIV

It has been suggested that there are two potential goals of NIV in ICU setting: to prevent ARF (preventive or prophylactic treatment), to treat ARF, and to avoid reintubation (curative treatment) [4]. Even if guidelines recommend not to use NIV in non-hypercapnic patients, NIV is used in 15% of ARDS patients worldwide [5]. Ventilator setting is a crucial point for NIV success. The total amount of pressure should not be higher than 15–20 cmH_2O. This pressure is the sum of positive end-expiratory pressure (PEEP) and pressure support (PS) used. PEEP will be used to avoid lung collapse and PS to increase tidal volume. Targeted tidal volume must be between 6 and 8 mL/kg of predicted body weight. Actual trends are high PEEP and low pressure support. If the total pressure is around 15 cmH_2O, the risk of gastric insufflation is low. NIV has been used after esophageal surgery, and the safety was correlated with the level of pressure used.

In spontaneously breathing patients, inspiration results in a negative pleural pressure, and a negative esophageal pressure, responsible of tidal volume. In pressure support, this negative pressure is the trigger of pressurization. Pressure support decreases work of breathing and the drive of mechanical ventilation. Thus, it decreases negative esophageal pressure. During acute respiratory failure, esophageal pressure in deeply negative and the transdiaphragmatic pressure may be positive increasing the risk of regurgitation. If pressure support ventilation (PSV) is efficient, esophageal pressure is less negative than in PSV. When the patient's drive is not decreased by PSV, with deep inspiration, even with low pressure support levels, the transpulmonary pressure increases, and the risk of gastric regurgitation remains high. The level of negative pressure, at the early inspiratory phase, is correlated to dyspnea. Thus, safety of enteral feeding must be discussed according to indication of NIV, curative or prophylactic.

9.4   Evaluation of Gastric Content

Risk of aspiration of gastric content is dependent of gastric content volume, a surrogate of enteral feeding tolerance. Gastric residual volume (GRV) measurement is not standardized or validated. Historically, gastric content was evaluated by gastric residual volume, aspired via the nasogastric tube using a 60 mL syringe. Although GRV monitoring was more accurate than physical examination and radiography for detecting gastrointestinal intolerance to EN, the accuracy of gastric aspiration for GRV measurement may vary according to tube position and diameter, number of tube openings, level of aspiration in the stomach, and experience of the evaluator.

Pulmonary aspiration of gastric contents is one of the most feared complications of anesthesia, which was reported to be one of the first causes of mortality related to general anesthesia. One of the risk factors for the occurrence of pulmonary aspiration and mainly for the onset of its clinical consequences is the volume of the aspirated gastric content [6]. Ultrasonographic examination of the gastric antrum is a noninvasive tool that has been described for preoperative assessment of gastric content and volume in both adults and children. This examination allowed the diagnosis of risk stomach, as defined by the presence of solid particles and/or a gastric fluid volume greater than 0.8 mL/kg before the induction of anesthesia, which could lead to symptomatic pulmonary aspiration of gastric contents in cases of regurgitation [7]. More recently, the same group showed that ultrasonographic examination of the antrum allowed for detection of gastric insufflation during preoxygenation of patient before elective surgery [8]. This simple examination, feasible in most ICU, allowed to recognize the stomach with low or high volume content and if facemask insufflation was responsible, or not, of gastric insufflation (Fig. 9.1). In their study, a peak airway pressure of 15 cmH_2O provided a probability of occurrence of gastric insufflation of

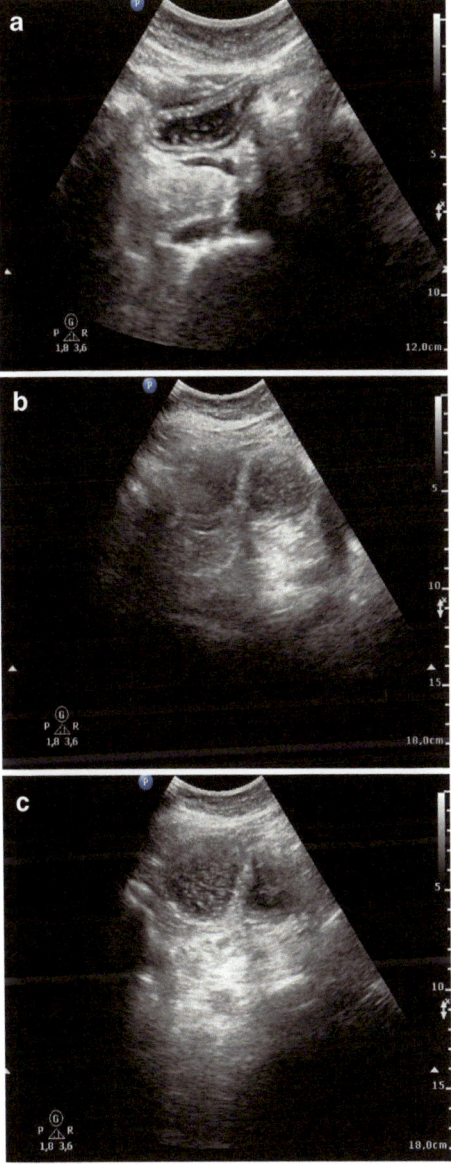

FIGURE 9.1 Example of gastric ultrasonographic images. (**a**) Normal gastric content. (**b**) Full gastric content. Antral cross-sectional area >400 mm². (**c**) Gastric insufflation with typical aspect of comets tail

35% according to real-time ultrasonography while providing the highest probability of acceptable facemask ventilation. This pressure limit was recommended for nonobese and non-paralyzed patients during pressure-controlled facemask ventilation in sedated patients. Furthermore, real-time ultrasonography of the antrum allowed for detection of gastric insufflation with high sensitivity; particularly, it detected entry of air into the stomach for low inspiratory pressures applied during ventilation. An obvious limitation to the application of these conclusions to patients receiving NIV is that all patients were sedated. Nevertheless, this level is comparable to levels recommended for NIV in ICU.

9.5   NIV and Enteral Feeding

Even if no data can recommend the use of ultrasonographic measurement of antral area, it can be an interesting tool for managing enteral feeding in patients receiving NIV. We can recommend a pragmatic approach depending of the timing of initiation of NIV and enteral feeding. Should "I" start NIV in this patient receiving enteral feeding, or should "I" initiate enteral feeding for this other patient receiving NIV? We decided to dichotomize according to the indication of NIV, curative or prophylactic.

For patients receiving NIV (Fig. 9.2), the first question is the indication:

1. If NIV is used as a prophylactic treatment, to avoid acute respiratory failure, we proposed to check gastric content. Antrum area assessed by ultrasonography is probably the most interesting way, but aspiration of gastric content may be used. This is true throughout the two algorithms. If gastric content is empty, initiating enteral feeding seems possible. We just recommend to check two times a day gastric content. In case of significant gastric content volume and antral cross-sectional area of 400 mm^2, air insufflation into the stomach during the NIV procedure is a major issue. If no sign of gastric insufflation is present, we recommend to

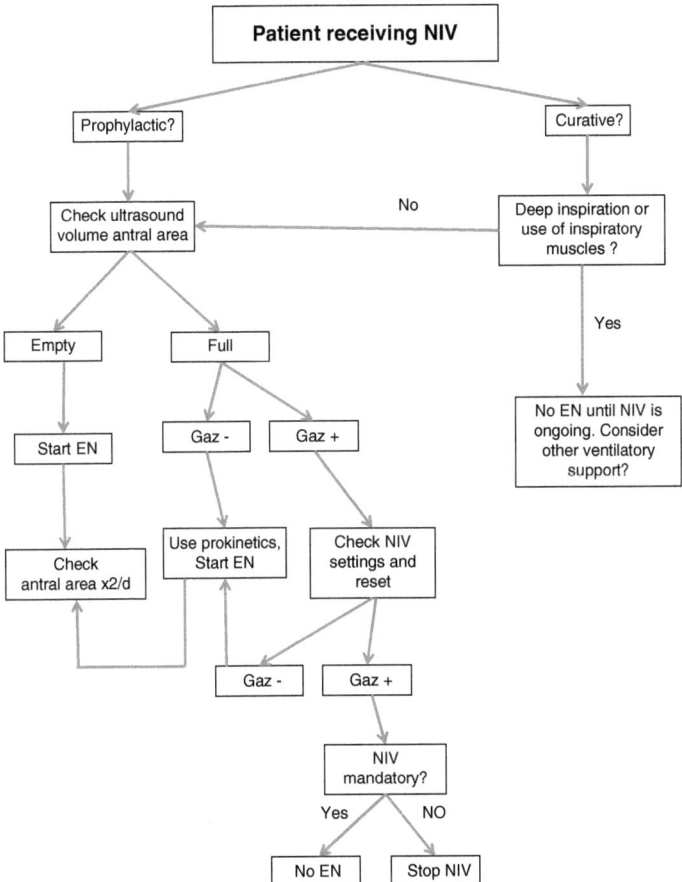

FIGURE 9.2 Algorithm for management of enteral nutrition (EN) for a patient receiving noninvasive ventilation (NIV). Gastric content is considered empty if antral CSA < 300 mm^2 and full if >400 mm^2. Between these two cutoffs, no clear recommendation could be done

start EN after initiation of prokinetics. If air insufflation is detected, we recommend to check ventilator setting, to decrease pressure support and/or PEEP, according to tidal volume, and recheck gastric content. If air disappears, start EN after prokinetics. If gastric insufflation is still ongoing, we think it is not safe to start enteral feeding. Physicians must consider other nutritional supports if NIV is mandatory or change ventilator support for high-flow nasal oxygen or continuous positive airway pressure.

2. If NIV is used as curative, to avoid intubation, the efforts done by the patients such as deep inspiration with the use of accessory inspiratory muscles and high transpulmonary pressure must be looked for. If such signs are present, we recommend not to start enteral feeding until the signs of distress or invasive ventilation have resolved. If NIV has decreased signs of ARF, without deep inspiration we think we can manage enteral feeding as we proposed for prophylactic NIV.

For patients receiving enteral feeding (Fig. 9.3), the first question should be "is NIV mandatory?" Physicians have to keep in mind that recent trials published on NIV are really challenging and the question must be answered carefully. Notwithstanding, if the answer is yes, the next step is curative or prophylactic. For prophylactic indications, according to gastric content, NIV might be started immediately or after initiation of prokinetics. In case NIV is used for curative indication and if the stomach is empty, initiation of NIV is acceptable. If the stomach is full, we recommend to start prokinetics and recheck. If gastric content is >300 mL, or antral $CSA > 400$ mm^2, NIV should not be started, and other ventilator supports, invasive or not, should be recommended. If gastric content decreases after prokinetics, NIV could be started. If NIV is initiated, we recommend to check gastric content two times a day.

9.6   Place of Parenteral Nutrition in Patients on NIV

In all cases, if enteral nutrition is insufficient to achieve targeted calories input, or if enteral feeding is impossible, parenteral nutrition (full or complementary) should be considered according to initial nutritional status (COPD, cancer, surgery, etc.), catabolism, and inflammation (ARF, sepsis, etc.).

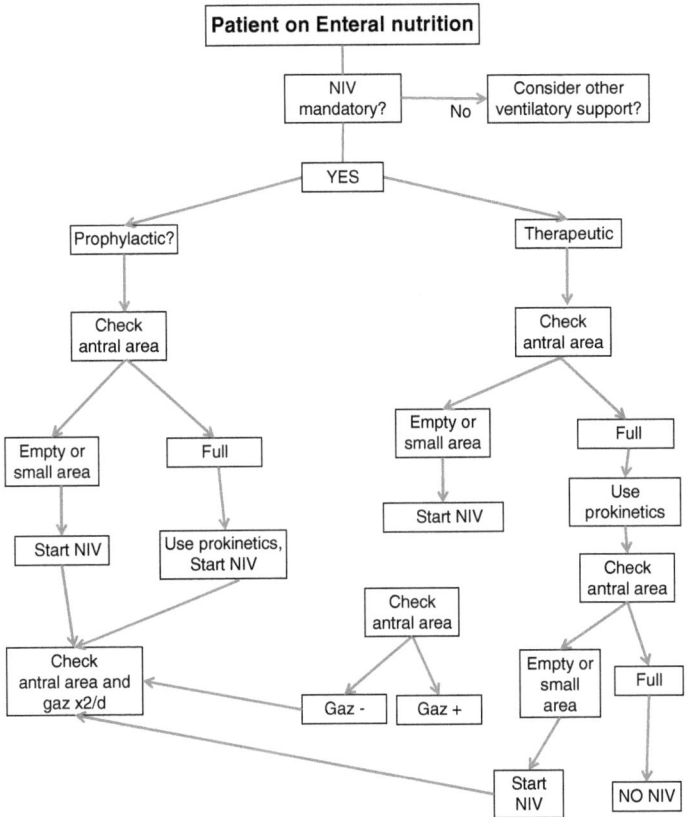

FIGURE 9.3 Algorithm for management of noninvasive ventilation (NIV) for a patient receiving enteral nutrition (EN)

9.7 Conclusion

Enteral feeding in patients receiving NIV, and vice versa, is not a casus belli. In patients receiving NIV for prophylactic indication, or for COPD patients without distress, checking gastric content and ventilator setting is mandatory but most often sufficient. As reported by Plant et al., in COPD patients, the non-delayed enteral feeding in medical ward does not increase complications [9]. When NIV is used for a patient in acute respiratory failure, physicians must be aware that NIV is not the Holy Grail even in specific patients such as the immunocompromised. In any cases, if used, NIV should be cautiously monitored. Gastric ultrasonography sounds like a promising technique that may help physicians in the management of these difficult situations.

References

1. Jaber S, Lescot T, Futier E, Paugam-Burtz C, Seguin P, Ferrandiere M, et al. NIVAS Study Group. Effect of noninvasive ventilation on tracheal reintubation among patients with hypoxemic respiratory failure following abdominal surgery. JAMA. 2016;315(13):1–9.
2. Preiser J-C, van Zanten ARH, Berger MM, Biolo G, Casaer MP, Doig GS, et al. Metabolic and nutritional support of critically ill patients: consensus and controversies. Crit Care. 2015;19(1):35.
3. Kogo M, Nagata K, Morimoto T, Ito J, Sato Y, Teraoka S, et al. Enteral nutrition is a risk factor for airway complications in subjects undergoing noninvasive ventilation for acute respiratory failure. Respir Care. 2017;62(4):459–67.
4. Demoule A, Chevret S, Carlucci A, Kouatchet A, Jaber S, Meziani F, et al. Changing use of noninvasive ventilation in critically ill patients: trends over 15 years in francophone countries. Intensive Care Med. 2015;42(1):82–92.
5. Bellani G, Laffey JG, Pham T, Fan E, Brochard L, Esteban A, et al. LUNG SAFE Investigators and the ESICM Trials Group. Epidemiology, patterns of care, and mortality for patients with acute respiratory distress syndrome in intensive care units in 50 countries. JAMA. 2016;315(8):788–13.
6. Lienhart A, Auroy Y, Péquignot F, Benhamou D, Warszawski J, Bovet M, Jougla E. Survey of anesthesia-related mortality in France. Anesthesiology. 2006;105(6):1087–97.
7. Bouvet L, Mazoit J-X, Chassard D, Allaouchiche B, Boselli E, Benhamou D. Clinical assessment of the ultrasonographic measurement of antral area for estimating preoperative gastric content and volume. Anesthesiology. 2011;114(5):1086–92.

8. Bouvet L, Albert M-L, Augris C, Boselli E, Ecochard R, Rabilloud M, Chassard D, Allaouchiche B. Real-time detection of gastric insufflation related to facemask pressure-controlled ventilation using ultrasonography of the antrum and epigastric auscultation in nonparalyzed patients: a prospective, randomized, double-blind study. Anesthesiology. 2014;120(2):326–34.
9. Plant PK, Owen JL, Elliott MW. Early use of non-invasive ventilation for acute exacerbations of chronic obstructive pulmonary disease on general respiratory wards: a multicentre randomised controlled trial. Lancet. 2000;355(9219):1931–5.

Chapter 10
The Very Old Patient

Luboš Sobotka

10.1 Introduction

There is significant prolongation of average life expectancy of population, which is associated with increased mental and physical capacity and quality of life of older people. At present time very old patients are no more patients aged more than 65; very old patients are defined as being aged more than 80 years. This positive trend has two consequences for specialists, who are working in intensive care:

- The number of older patients, who undergo aggressive therapeutic procedure (surgical procedures, endoscopic or endovascular interventions), is growing. Indeed more advanced therapeutic procedures (e.g. endovascular interventions, laparoscopic surgery, joint replacement) have become accessible also for older patients.
- The proportion of older patients, who are hospitalized in ICU, is increasing. This is a result of extended age but also of more intensive treatment of very old patients.

L. Sobotka
3rd Department of Medicine Metabolic Care and
Gerontology, Medical Fakulty - Charles University in Prague,
Hradec Kralove, 50005, Czech Republic
e-mail: pustik@lfhk.cuni.cz

© Springer International Publishing AG 2018
M.M. Berger (ed.), *Critical Care Nutrition Therapy for Non-nutritionists*, https://doi.org/10.1007/978-3-319-58652-6_10

The major problem is that in spite of the fact that more elderly survive complicated medical intervention and subsequent stay and treatment in ICU, the full recovery of physical and psychic functions is less effective. Quite often older patients survive complicated disease; however, after discharge from hospital, his or her quality of life is low and not up to the therapeutic effort and cost of treatment. Instead, the patients (especially after stay in an ICU) are fully dependent on the help of other persons (especially family members or personnel in institution line nursing homes). In this way sometimes, successful ICU treatment only prolongs subsequent long-term dying. The loss of independence of very old subjects after aggressive treatment and ICU stay is paramount problem of current health care.

10.2   Characteristics of the Very Old ICU Patient

Several specificities combine in the very old patient:

- *Polymorbidity and polymedication*—The combination of numerous (usually chronic) diseases is frequent in very old subjects. This is usually connected with chronic low-grade inflammation, which prevents muscle gain and decreases physical activity [1].
- *Limited body protein reserve*—The total mass of protein localized in skeletal muscle is low or even exhausted in very old patients [2]. This condition is known as sarcopenia of the elderly [3] and results from several factors: the combination of hormonal changes, chronic inflammation, undernutrition and reduced physical activity is of paramount importance. Especially reduced physical activity leads to loss muscle mass, which again causes loss of physical activity and leads to vicious cycle (loss of muscle mass, loss of activity, etc.). Therefore, the very old persons are often protein depleted before the ICU stay.
- *Stay in the ICU*—The reason for the treatment in ICU is always critical illness, which is accompanied by

inflammation, immobilization in recumbent position and regularly low food intake. Hence, the ICU stay leads to catabolic reaction with subsequent further loss of muscle protein and subsequently to loss of muscle function. This, in turn, decreases the rehabilitation capacity of the geriatric patient.

– *Difficult recovery and muscle mass gain* — Rehabilitation and regain of muscle mass are more difficult in older patients that in younger subjects. This is due to muscle weakness, polymorbidity (mentioned above), loss of appetite as well as psychological problems that are common in very old patients especially during serious disease and ICU stay (delirium, depression and dementia).

10.3   Assessment of Nutritional Status

Due to the above specificities, a dedicated nutrition screening tool has been validated called the Mini-Nutritional Assessment (MNA) tool in a short form [4, 5],which in addition to the NRS variables includes an assessment of neuropsychological problems (confusion), chewing and swallowing difficulties as well as mobility which heavily impact on the patients' capacity to feed themselves. But these informations are not always available in the ICU.

The older subjects lose muscle more easily than their younger companions do. Especially physical activity is declining with age and that, in turn, leads to loss of muscle mass. Moreover, each inflammatory response increases catabolism of muscle tissue, which normally serves as a source of substrates (especially amino acids) to tissues and organs, which are important for survival of acute illness. The presence of muscle protein stores and subsequent muscle catabolism during critical state are principally important for both inflammatory reaction and early immune response, as in other age categories.

Loss of muscle mass together with polymorbidity and psychological problems (dementia, delirium and depression) is responsible for the decreased effectivity of ICU treatment in very old patients. Such combination makes older patients extremely susceptible to any stress and is called frailty. In the frail patients, even a short ICU stay leads to critical depletion of muscle mass and immobility and subsequent complications (e.g. pressure sores). As muscle mass loss results from immobilization, inflammation and malnutrition, the subsequent rehabilitation and recovery of such old subjects are usually impossible.

Patient falls into cycle of inflammation with subsequent loss of appetite and immobilization accompanied with psychological problems such as depression and especially delirium. Particularly delirium is often treated by sedatives, which in turn decreases possibility for physiotherapy, rehabilitation and normal food intake. All these mechanisms lead to further muscle mass loss and escalation of vicious (futile) cycle; even if older patient survives acute illness, he or she is fully dependent and the life ends in nursing house.

10.4   Recommendations for Nutrition Support in Older Patients

Even well-nourished subject admitted to ICU immediately starts to lose the lean body mass and subsequently the muscle strength. The nutrition support plays an indispensable role in the treatment of such patients, because of anticipation that the loss of lean body mass including the muscles will be even worse after ICU stay. However, it must be always in harmony with treatment plan and medical procedures. The following recommendations are important:

10.4.1   Outcome-Based Approach

Determination of the realistic and accessible outcomes of the ICU treatment is important condition of the treatment of older subject. This is because very old subjects are at particular risk of loss of critical muscle mass and subsequent full dependence on medical treatment. Therefore, the ICU treatment plan including nutrition support must be dependent on scheduled outcomes. When the realistic treatment goal is the independent life after discharge from the hospital, then the complete therapeutic effort must focus on this outcome. Then precise nutrition must always be included into the treatment plans.

10.4.2   Early Realization of Nutritional Plan

As very old and often depleted or sarcopenic patient is at risk of treatment failure, the nutrition support must be commenced without any delay. The planned amount and composition of nutrition support are more important than the way of nutrient administration. The enteral nutrition is always preferable (Table 10.1); however, achieving the planned goals of nutrition support is the most important issue. Therefore, if the patient does not tolerate the planned nutrition via gastric or enteral tube, it is necessary to start with total or supplemental parenteral nutrition.

10.4.3   Nutrition Support Must Not Lead to Immobilization of the Patient

Insertion of nasogastric or nasojejunal tube in older patient is often associated with poor tolerance and spontaneous tube removal; it is rarely true for intravenous catheter. Therefore, some physicians and nurses use pharmacological sedation in order to prevent feeding tube removal. Nevertheless, sedatives prevent physical activity, and subsequent immobilization impairs important nutritional goal—muscle gain or, at least, an avoidance of muscle loss [6]. The tube feeding should be used only when well tolerated and does not prevent physical activity and rehabilitation therapy. If it is not possible, then parenteral nutrition and subsequent early oral feeding are indicated [7]. The feeding method should never be a reason for immobilization.

TABLE 10.1 Recommendations for ICU management of the old elderly

Aims and tools	General	Comment
Early nutritional plan	Enteral nutrition is always preferable Tube feeding should be used only when well tolerated Combined or pure parenteral may be required	Limit the use pharmacological sedation in order to prevent feeding tube removal Consider early percutaneous endoscopic gastrostomy (PEG)
Prevention of refeeding syndrome	Regular control of plasma potassium, phosphate and magnesium Systematic intake of these electrolytes is crucial	Frequent requirements: K > 2 mmol/kg*d P 0.5–0.7 mmol/kg*d Mg 0.2–0.3 mmol/kg of body weight
Monitoring	Real daily intakes	Diarrhoea: stool volume < 300 ml/day
Prevention of immobilization	Early physical programme	

10.4.4   Control of Nutritional Goals and Absorption

It was shown that real intake of nutrients using enteral nutrition (sipping and especially tube feeding) is usually lower than planned. This is often due to reduced tolerance and side effects as well as due to therapeutic and diagnostic procedures or gut problems secondary to critical illness. In addition, loss of energy in the stool can be significant; in ICU patients, the energy loss via stool reached more than 300 kcal/day during enteral nutrition [8].

10.4.5   Prevention of Refeeding Syndrome

As very old patients can be undernourished and depleted, the full nutrition support can lead to development of refeeding syndrome. Especially when inflammatory process ceases and anabolism is imminent, there is great risk of complications, which are consequences of refeeding syndrome [9]. Mainly muscle weakness, paraesthesia and cramps together with arrhythmias and heart failure are common consequences, but also episodes of confusion.

10.5   The Goals of Nutrition Support

Regarding to the composition of nutrients, there is no substantial difference between middle-aged and very old ICU patients [10]. However, there are some aspects that should be highlighted (see Table 10.2).

The recommended intake of energy will depend on scheduled goals of nutrition support, especially for healing process and for physical activity important for muscle mass gain. According to some measurements, the physical activity during rehabilitation therapy is associated with increased energy expenditure 50% more energy than basic energy expenditure. This corresponds to the intake of 37–45 kcal per kg and day [11, 12].

If the goal is to achieve positive protein balance, then supplementary protein must be part of nutrition support. If measured energy expenditure is the basis for nutrition support [13], consider delivering particularly high proportions of pro-

TABLE 10.2 Nutritional targets

	Target	**Comment**
Energy	Early: 20–25 kcal/kg of body weight/day Recovery: 37–45 kcal kg/day	Rehabilitation requirements are frequently underestimated
Protein	1.5–2.0 g/kg/day	Protein-rich oral supplements may be required

teins/amino acids, as they are building blocks for regenerated tissue: protein-rich oral nutrition supplements are a practical way to increase the part of proteins in total energy intake.

10.6   Importance of Extended Nutrition Support

It is difficult or even impossible to maintain any critically ill patient in positive or even in zero protein balance. The very old patient is no exception; in fact older patients treated in the ICU have less functional muscle mass. The recovery and related increase of muscle mass are more difficult in old and sarcopenic subjects than in middle-aged patients. Therefore, nutrition management must be an essential part of treatment; this is important especially during period of healing and recovery and also during rehabilitation period.

The nutrition goals should be significantly higher than basic energy expenditure in very old patient during convalescence period. There are no clinical trials supporting general recommendations in the group of older patients treated in the ICU. However, we have shown that combination of nutrition support and early physical activity led to significant improvement of psychical activity after severe acute illness in very old patients [14]. The composition and combination of nutritional substrates should be planned on outcome-based estimations. If the goal on nutrition support is to increase muscle mass and hence the muscle function, which was lost during ICU stay, then the amount and composition of nutritional substrates should be more pro anabolic. However, without physical activity ingested substrates (especially fat) are stored in adipose tissue.

References

1. Lightfoot AP, McCormick R, Nye GA, McArdle A. Mechanisms of skeletal muscle ageing; avenues for therapeutic intervention. Curr Opin Pharmacol. 2014;16:116–21.

2. Pirlich M, Schutz T, Norman K, et al. The German hospital malnutrition study. Clin Nutr. 2006;25:563–72.
3. Morley JE. Sarcopenia in the elderly. Fam Pract. 2012; 29(Suppl 1):i44–i8.
4. Bauer JM, Vogl T, Wicklein S, Trogner J, Muhlberg W, Sieber CC. Comparison of the mini nutritional assessment, subjective global assessment, and nutritional risk screening (NRS 2002) for nutritional screening and assessment in geriatric hospital patients. Z Gerontol Geriatr. 2005;38:322–7.
5. Volkert D, Berner YN, Berry E, et al. ESPEN guidelines on enteral nutrition: geriatrics. Clin Nutr. 2006;25:330–60.
6. Cohen S, Nathan JA, Goldberg AL. Muscle wasting in disease: molecular mechanisms and promising therapies. Nat Rev Drug Discov. 2015;14:58–74.
7. Sobotka L, Schneider SM, Berner YN, et al. ESPEN guidelines on parenteral nutrition: geriatrics. Clin Nutr. 2009;28:461–6.
8. Strack van Schijndel RJ, Wierdsma NJ, van Heijningen EM, Weijs PJ, de Groot SD, Girbes AR. Fecal energy losses in enterally fed intensive care patients: an explorative study using bomb calorimetry. Clin Nutr. 2006;25:758–64.
9. Friedli N, Stanga Z, Sobotka L, et al. Revisiting the refeeding syndrome: results of a systematic review. Nutrition. 2017;35:151–60.
10. Segadilha NL, Rocha EE, Tanaka LM, Gomes KL, Espinoza RE, Peres WA. Energy expenditure in critically ill elderly patients: indirect calorimetry vs predictive equations. JPEN J Parenter Enteral Nutr. 2016;41:776–784.
11. Poehlman ET. Energy expenditure and requirements in aging humans. J Nutr. 1992;122:2057–65.
12. Poehlman ET, Arciero PJ, Goran MI. Endurance exercise in aging humans: effects on energy metabolism. Exerc Sport Sci Rev. 1994;22:251–84.
13. Zusman O, Theilla M, Cohen J, Kagan I, Bendavid I, Singer P. Resting energy expenditure, calorie and protein consumption in critically ill patients: a retrospective cohort study. Crit Care. 2016;20:367.
14. Hegerova P, Dedkova Z, Sobotka L. Early nutritional support and physiotherapy improved long-term self-sufficiency in acutely ill older patients. Nutrition. 2015;31:166–70.

Chapter 11
Inborn Errors of Metabolism in Adults: Clues for Nutritional Management in ICU

Christel Tran and Luisa Bonafé

11.1 Introduction

Inborn errors of metabolism (IEM) result from the absence or abnormality of an enzyme or its cofactor, leading to the accumulation or deficiency of a specific metabolite. Approximately 500 human diseases due to IEMs are recognized. This number is increasing as novel techniques become available and allow for the identification of new biochemical and molecular abnormalities [1]. IEM are individually rare; however, taken together they affect about 1 in 1000 to 1 in 4500 people [2]. Majority of the disease are pediatric; however, with the identification of late-onset forms and with improved survival, they are conditions that must be considered in patients of all ages. Improved prognosis of children with IEM has significantly increased the number of adult

C. Tran (✉) • L. Bonafé
Division of Genetic Medicine, Center for Molecular Diseases,
Lausanne University Hospital, Lausanne, Switzerland
e-mail: Christel.Tran@chuv.ch

© Springer International Publishing AG 2018   133
M.M. Berger (ed.), *Critical Care Nutrition Therapy*
for Non-nutritionists, https://doi.org/10.1007/978-3-319-58652-6_11

patients with these conditions, and specialized ICU should be aware of the risks and pitfalls of managing them.

Acute metabolic decompensation of IEM may be induced by catabolic triggers such as critical illness, fasting, infection, and surgery making ICU a risk area for patients with IEM. IEM susceptible to suffer metabolic decompensation necessitating specific nutritional management are summarized in Fig. 11.1 and can be divided into two main categories: (1) disorders that

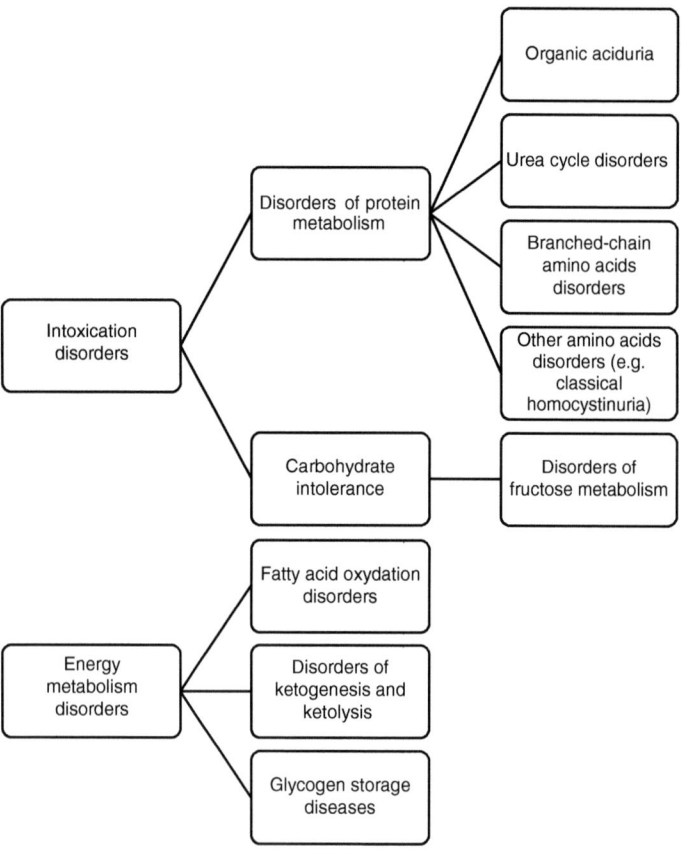

FIGURE 11.1 Examples of inborn errors of metabolism in adults susceptible to metabolic decompensation and specific nutritional management

give rise to intoxication (this group includes IEM that lead to an acute or progressive intoxication from the accumulation of toxic compound proximal to the metabolic block) and (2) disorders associated with energy deficiency that consist of IEM with symptoms due mainly to a deficiency in energy production (primary mitochondrial energy disorders) or utilization (disorders of glycogenolysis and gluconeogenesis). Manifestation can be as a late-onset features of a complex multisystemic disease, but sometimes it can also be the only manifestation of an underlying IEM (Fig. 11.1). This chapter relates IEM that may be responsible for life-threatening conditions in adulthood and require a particular nutritional management.

11.2   Specific Metabolic Characteristics

In this section, we discuss examples of IEM and their main clinical and biological characteristics.

11.2.1   Intoxication Disorders

Deficiencies of enzymes involved in amino acid metabolism frequently result in accumulation of toxic substances and subsequent organ damage. The brain, liver, and kidneys are the most frequently affected organs. Acute symptoms are often associated with catabolic states that lead to the breakdown of endogenous protein and the release of large amounts of amino acids. The clinical feature results from the toxicity of the accumulating metabolites and concurrent product deficiency; they depend on the severity of the enzyme deficiency and the extent of the protein intake or endogenous amino acid release in protein catabolism. Typical features of metabolic decompensation include coma, encephalopathy, progressive neurologic symptoms, and unclear deterioration of the patient. Hyperammonemia, metabolic acidosis, elevated lactate, and ketosis are common findings. Adult-onset clinical presentation can present for the first time with a metabolic decompensation triggered by an event such as major surgery, fever, and unusual low or high protein load intake (fasting presurgery, parenteral nutrition) [3, 4]. Therefore, measurement of ammonia profile should always be considered in adults presenting with catabolic stressors and (1) unexplained acute encephalopathy, (2) unusual or unexplained neurological illness, (3) liver failure, and/or (4) suspected intoxication. If hyperammonemia is confirmed, determination of plasma amino acids, acylcarnitine, urine organic, and orotic acid should be urgently requested together with basic laboratory investigations, not waiting for the results (which should be obtained in <24 h) for treating the patient. Alteration of arginine, lysine, ornithine, and citrulline levels associated with elevated urinary orotic acid will be highly suggestive of urea cycle disorders, whereas elevated organic acids or acylcarnitine may orientate the diagnosis toward organic aciduria or fatty acid oxidation disorders.

11.2.2   Disorders Associated with Energy Deficiency

Mitochondrial fatty acid oxidation (FAO) represents an important pathway for energy production during situations that result in increased demand such as fasting, febrile illness, and muscular exertion. Insufficient ketone body production due to impaired β-oxidation in combination with inhibition of gluconeogenesis by low acetyl-CoA during catabolic stress (prolonged fasting, surgery, infection) may present with three typical features: (1) acute hypoketotic hypoglycemia, with encephalopathy, hepatomegaly, and liver dysfunction, (2) cardiomyopathy and arrhythmia, and (3) myopathy with myalgia and rhabdomyolysis. Adult-onset presentation is also typically precipitated by metabolic stressors [5]. Basic biochemistry analysis for FAO includes glucose, ammonia, lactate, blood gas, transaminases, creatine kinase (CK), and urinary ketones. The key investigation analysis is acylcarnitine profiling where accumulation of specific acyl-CoAs chains (short, medium, or long) will be diagnostic. Overall, specific biochemistry investigations for IEM should be carried out by a specialist metabolic biochemistry laboratory and interpretation by a metabolic specialist.

Glycogen storage disease type I (von Gierke disease) is an inborn error of carbohydrate metabolism and mainly affects glycogenolysis and gluconeogenesis. During metabolic decompensation, glycogen degradation pyruvate and lactate results increase lipogenesis and production of uric acid which give rise to lactic academia, hyperlipidemia, and hyperuricemia, respectively. The main goal of treatment for liver GSDs is to maintain normoglycemia and suppress secondary metabolic derangements by ensuring regular carbohydrate intake. Long-term complications of GSD I include liver adenomas, renal insufficiency, and gout attacks [6].

11.3   Nutritional Characteristics and Timing of Nutritional Intervention

The primary goal of the dietary therapy of decompensated IEM is to prevent worsening of catabolism and improve metabolic control through adaptation of protein, fat, and carbohydrate intake according to the type of metabolism involved.

11.3.1   Intoxication Disorders

The long-term management of aminoacidopathies is aimed at decreasing the accumulation of the toxic amino acid and is specific for each disease [4, 7–9]. In general, protein restriction plus a semisynthetic amino acid supplement that does not contain the accumulating amino acids is recommended as well as supplementation of minerals, trace elements, and sometimes essential fatty acid. Beware of protein deficiency due to "overtreatment" which may cause protein catabolism and triggers the metabolic decompensation. During metabolic decompensation and according to its severity, protein intake may initially be stopped (for no more than 24 h) and intravenous (IV) glucose started (Table 11.1). The aim is to prevent endogenous catabolism, in particular protein catabolism, while providing enough calories to meet metabolic demands. Insulin can be carefully used to promote anabolism while maintaining normoglycemia. Supplementation with essential amino acids (particularly branched chain amino acids) will also enhance anabolism without excessive nitrogen load [10]. Monitoring of lactate is recommended during IV glucose due to potential interference with Krebs cycle entry and inhibition of pyruvate dehydrogenase by toxic metabolites. Lipid emulsion may provide additional calories [4]. Specific detoxifying drugs (e.g., in urea cycle defects, organic aciduria) and/or specific vitamins, or cofactors (e.g., in classical homocystinuria) can be used. L-Carnitine is given in organic aciduria to compensate for secondary carnitine deficiency caused by urinary loss of carnitine-bound to organic acids [7]. It is essential to start treatment without delay as the accumulation of toxic amino acid, substrate, and/ or ammonia can be devastating for the patient and eventually fatal. In severe decompensation, toxic metabolites may also be removed by hemodiafiltration.

11.3.2   Disorders Associated with Energy Deficiency

Prolonged fasting (>24 h) should be avoided in all FAO disorders (FAOD) to reduce the risk of acute decompensation. Long-chain fat is restricted in patients with severe long-chain FAOD such as very-long-chain acyl-CoA dehydrogenase (VLCAD) deficiency. Replacement medium-chain fats are used as they can enter the mitochondria independently of carnitine and bypass the long-chain beta-oxidation enzymes. Triheptanoin is an ester of three C7 fatty acids and is thought to be more effective than medium-chain triglycerides (MCT). A phase 2 clinical study is currently underway (www.clinicaltrials.gov, NCT01379625). Some adults may follow a normal diet when well, but dietary modifications (with IV glucose if needed) may be advisable during periods of metabolic stress such as intercurrent illness or surgery [11]. The aim is to provide sufficient glucose to stimulate insulin secretion and suppression of lipolysis. Hypoglycemia in an adult patient with an FAOD is a late event, and additional glucose should be started without delay before the blood glucose falls.

TABLE 11.1 Examples of IEM potentially requiring urgent dietary treatment in adulthood

Disease group	Disease name examples	Metabolic decompensation	Nutritional management
INTOXICATION DISORDERS			
UCD	CPS1 deficiency OTC Citrullinemia types 1 and 2 Argininosuccinic aciduria Argininemia HHH syndrome	Hyperammonemia Perturbation of AA profile (citrulline, ornithine, arginine) ↑ Urine orotate	– Stop protein during 24–48 h – EAA formula – Natural protein reintroduction (0.8 g/kg/day)[a] when NH3 level < 100 µmol/L – IV glucose (3–4 mg/kg/min) – ±Insulin (initial 0.01–0.02 UI/kg/h) – Lipid emulsion (up to 2 g/kg/day) – L-Arginine[b] – Vitamins, minerals supplementation
BCAAD	MSUD	AA profile: ↑ leucine, isoleucine, valine and alloisoleucine	– BCAA-free proteins – Glucose and insulin perfusion (same as UCD) – Early isoleucine and valine supplementation[c] – Reintroduction of intact protein when Leucine <300 µmol/L

(continued)

Table 11.1 (continued)

Disease group	Disease name examples	Metabolic decompensation	Nutritional management
OA	PA MMA	Metabolic acidosis, ketosis, hyperammonemia, lactic acidosis, hypoglycemia OA in urine: ↑BCAA metabolite	– Same as UCD[b] – IV carnitine (increase to 100–200 mg/kg/day) – Bicarbonate if acidosis
Classical homocystinuria	Classical homocystinuria	↑ Plasma Hcy and met level	– Restriction of met intake (met-free EAA mixture)[d] – Protein (0.83 g/kg/day)[a] – Vitamin B6, folate, vitamin B12[d] – ±Oral betaine (max 3 g twice daily)

DISORDERS INVOLVING ENERGY METABOLISM

FAOD	MCAD VLCAD LCHAD SCAD CPT1A CPT2 CDSP CACT } D	Hypoketotic hypoglycemia, ↑CK, ± lactic acidosis OA: Dicarboxylic aciduria	– Prevention of hypoglycemia (Bolus: 2ml/kg of 10% glucose then maintenance for glucose requirement 3–4 mg/kg/min) – ±Carnitine supplementation (50–100 mg/kg/day if plasma concentrations are low) – MCTs in VLCAD
Disorder of ketogenesis	HMG-Coa synthase deficiency	Same as FAOD	– Same as in FAOD
Disorders of ketolysis	SCOT B-ketothiolase deficiency	Ketoacidosis (rare after 10 years of age) OA: ↑2-methyl-3-hydroxybutyrate, tiglylglycine	Same as in FAOD – Bicarbonate if acidosis

(continued)

TABLE 11.1 (continued)

Disease group	Disease name examples	Metabolic decompensation	Nutritional management
GSD I	Liver GSD (I, III, IV, VI, IX, XI) Muscle GSD (II and V)	GSD I: Hypoglycemia, ↑ lactate, ↑ uric acid, ↑ triglycerides, lactic acidosis	– Maintaining blood glucose levels ≥70 mg/dL – Avoid fasting more than 5–6 h – IV glucose if oral and enteral feeding not tolerated: Bolus: 2ml/kg of 10% glucose. Then maintenance for glucose requirement 3–4 mg/kg/min[e] – Bicarbonate if acidosis – Vitamins, mineral supplementation

AA amino acid, *EAA* essential amino acid, *BCAAD* branched-chain amino acid deficiency, *CACT* carnitine acylcarnitine translocase, *CDSP* systemic primary carnitine deficiency, *CPT* carnitine palmitoyltransferase 1, *D* deficiency, *FAOD* Fatty acid oxidation disorders, *GSD* glycogen storage disease, *Hcy* homocysteine, *HHH* hyperammonemia, hyperornithinemia, homocitrullinemia, *IV* intravenous, *LCHAD* long-chain hydroxyacyl-CoA dehydrogenase deficiency, *MCAD* medium-chain acyl-CoA dehydrogenase deficiency, *MCT* medium-chain triglycerides, *Met* methionine, *MMA* methylmalonic aciduria, *OA* organic acid, *OTC* ornithine transcarbamylase, *PA* propionic aciduria, *SCAD* short-chain acyl-CoA dehydrogenase deficiency, *SCOT* succinyl-CoA3-oxoacid CoA transferase, *UCD* urea cycle disorders, *VLCAD* very long-chain acyl-CoA dehydrogenase deficiency

[a]Selected values from FAO/WHO/UNU for safe levels of protein intake [4]

[b]Dose according to specific guidelines [4, 7]

[c]Dose according to specific guideline [9]

[d]Dose according to specific guideline [8]

[e]Dose according to specific guideline [6]

11.4 Specific Needs of the Category and Feeding Route

11.4.1 Intoxication Disorders

Enteral route is to be preferred whenever not contraindicated. There is ample evidence that enteral protein intake is advantageous over parenteral amino acid intake in promoting anabolism [10]. Moreover it should be remembered that it is possible to provide more energy and nutrients in a smaller volume through enteral feeds than via parenteral nutrition (PN). But if there are contraindications, the parenteral route is valuable. However PN should be used very carefully in certain conditions where specific amino acids intake should be limited (e.g., methionine in classical homocystinuria, leucine in maple syrup urine disease, phenylalanine in phenylketonuria). PN solutions are not necessarily adjusted for patients with decompensated IEM of amino acid metabolism, and suitable solutions must indeed be prepared. This preparation needs a close collaboration between the ICU physician, the metabolic specialist, and the pharmacy [12]. During acute metabolic decompensation, an amino acid-free parenteral solution is suitable for the first 24–48 h, but protein must then be added using commercially available standard amino acid solutions (containing essential and nonessential amino acids). Initially, amino acids are introduced in an amount sufficient to meet safe levels of protein intake and then titrated according to biochemical monitoring of amino acids. Vitamins, minerals, and micronutrients must always be provided to prevent selective deficiencies.

11.4.2 Disorders Associated with Energy Deficiency

PN should also be used cautiously in FAO and fructose disorders. In the late 1960s, deleterious effects of high-dose IV fructose were also recognized in healthy persons.

Hyperuricemia [13] and lactic acidosis [14] were the prominent findings and are due to the influence of fructose on purine catabolism and glycolytic pathway, respectively. These observations have led to the recommendation of great caution when using fructose in PN [15]. IV lipid should not be given in FAOD and ketogenesis disorders. Medium-chain triglycerides (MCTs) can be given via NG tube or G tube to proven disorders of long-chain fatty acid oxidation and the carnitine cycle because of their rapid and complete oxidation. However, they are contraindicated in patients with MCAD and HMG-CoA synthase deficiency as they may accumulate in the plasma (MCAD guidelines: bimdg.org.uk\guidelines). In patients with severe FAOD, overnight fasting may need to be avoided and managed with uncooked cornstarch or continuous overnight pump feeding.

In GSD I, frequent supply of exogenous glucose must be maintained during catabolic triggers (e.g., fasting >5 h, fever) using glucose polymer drinks or IV glucose if enteral route is not tolerated (Table 11.1).

11.5   Monitoring of the Intervention

11.5.1   Intoxication Disorders

Close monitoring of the toxic substances is needed until the values are within the recommended target. Regular laboratory monitoring of patients on protein-restricted diet should include blood count, calcium, phosphate, magnesium, iron, liver, kidney function tests, alkaline phosphatase, total protein, albumin, pre-albumin, vitamin B12, cholesterol, triglycerides, vitamins, carnitine, acid-base status, ammonia, lactate, amino acids in plasma, and organic acids in urine.

Following improvement of metabolic and clinical abnormalities, natural protein preferably, should be reintroduced rapidly with the aim of meeting safe levels of protein intake (Table 11.1) and not withheld more than 24(−48) h.

11.5.2   Disorders Associated with Energy Deficiency

Biochemical follow-up of FAOD includes monitoring of glucose, free carnitine and acylcarnitines, CK, and transaminases. Free carnitine is measured to monitor carnitine supplementation in patients with primary carnitine deficiency [16]. Except if plasma carnitine levels are severely decreased, carnitine supplementation is not currently recommended in other FAOD. Carnitine supplementation may even be detrimental in disorders of long-chain fatty acid oxidation of the carnitine cycle, due to the cardiotoxicity of the long-chain acylcarnitines.

Regarding GSD I, when metabolic control is achieved (stable glucose level $\geq$ 70 mg/dL) and enteral route tolerated, frequent meals can be provided (nutrient distribution: 60–70% carbohydrate, 10–15% protein, <30% fat). Good glucose control can help prevent the long-term complications of GSD I.

11.6   Conclusion

The aim of this chapter was to provide the reader with information on how to initiate nutritional therapy in main IEM disorders susceptible to have a metabolic decompensation and be admitted to the ICU. Adequate nutritional therapy is often essential to the good prognosis of these patients and requires special attention in terms of specific management and follow-up.

References

1. Childs B, Kinzler KW, Vogelstein B, editors. The Metabolic and Molecular Bases of Inherited Disease. 8th edn. McGraw-Hill, New York, 2001.
2. Das SK. Inborn Errors of Metabolism: Challenges and Management. Indian J Clin Biochem. 2013;28(4): 311–3.

3. Cavicchi C, Donati M, Parini R, Rigoldi M, Bernardi M, Orfei F, Gentiloni Silveri N, Colasante A, Funghini S, Catarzi S, et al. Sudden unexpected fatal encephalopathy in adults with OTC gene mutations-clues for early diagnosis and timely treatment. Orphanet J Rare Dis. 2014;9:105.
4. Joint WHO/FAO/UNU Expert Consultation. Protein and amino acid requirements in human nutrition. World Health Organ Tech Rep Ser. 2007;935:1–265.
5. Lang TF. Adult presentations of medium-chain acyl-CoA dehydrogenase deficiency (MCADD). J Inherit Metab Dis. 2009;32(6):675–83.
6. Kishnani PS, Austin SL, Abdenur JE, Arn P, Bali DS, Boney A, Chung WK, Dagli AI, Dale D, Koeberl D, et al. Diagnosis and management of glycogen storage disease type I: a practice guideline of the American College of Medical Genetics and Genomics. Genet Med. 2014;16(11):e1.
7. Baumgartner MR, Horster F, Dionisi-Vici C, Haliloglu G, Karall D, Chapman KA, Huemer M, Hochuli M, Assoun M, Ballhausen D, et al. Proposed guidelines for the diagnosis and management of methylmalonic and propionic acidemia. Orphanet J Rare Dis. 2014;9:130.
8. Morris AA, Kozich V, Santra S, Andria G, Ben-Omran TI, Chakrapani AB, Crushell E, Henderson MJ, Hochuli M, Huemer M, et al. Guidelines for the diagnosis and management of cystathionine beta-synthase deficiency. J Inherit Metab Dis. 2017;40(1):49–74.
9. Frazier DM, Allgeier C, Homer C, Marriage BJ, Ogata B, Rohr F, Splett PL, Stembridge A, Singh RH. Nutrition management guideline for maple syrup urine disease: an evidence- and consensus-based approach. Mol Genet Metab. 2014;112(3):210–7.
10. Boneh A. Dietary protein in urea cycle defects: how much? Which? How? Mol Genet Metab. 2014;113(1–2):109–12.
11. Spiekerkoetter U, Lindner M, Santer R, Grotzke M, Baumgartner MR, Boehles H, Das A, Haase C, Hennermann JB, Karall D, et al. Treatment recommendations in long-chain fatty acid oxidation defects: consensus from a workshop. J Inherit Metab Dis. 2009;32(4):498–505.
12. Tran C, Luisa B, Nuoffer JM, Rieger J, Berger MM. Adult classical homocystinuria requiring parenteral nutrition: Pitfalls and management. Clin Nutr. 2017. e-pub 25 July, doi: 10.1016/j.clnu.2017.07.013.
13. Perheentupa J, Raivio K. Fructose-induced hyperuricaemia. Lancet. 1967;2(7515):528–31.

14. Bergstrom J, Hultman E, Roch-Norlund AE. Lactic acid accu-
    mulation in connection with fructose infusion. Acta Med Scand.
    1968;184(5):359–64.
15. Tran C. Inborn errors of fructose metabolism. What can we learn
    from them. Forum Nutr. 2017;9(4).
16. Magoulas PL, et al. Systemic primary carnitine deficiency: an
    overview of clinical manifestations, diagnosis, and management.
    Orphanet J Rare Dis. 2012;7:68.

Chapter 12
Chronic Critical Illness

Michael A. Via and Jeffrey I. Mechanick

12.1 Introduction

Patients who survive an acute severe medical insult but who continue to require intensive medical care enter into a state of chronic critical illness (CCI). Nonadaptive molecular and cellular responses render CCI as a unique condition, without evolutionary precedent, that is only possible through modern medical practices [1].

Once the CCI state is reached, clinically significant improvements become far more difficult. Strategies of supportive care, including nutrition support, should be implemented to mitigate the extreme stress of allostatic overload in CCI.

M.A. Via (✉) • J.I. Mechanick*
Division of Endocrinology, Diabetes, and Bone Disease, Mount Sinai Beth Israel Medical Center, Icahn School of Medicine at Mount Sinai, New York, NY, USA
e-mail: michael.via@mountsinai.org

*The Marie-Josee and Henry R. Kravis Center for Cardiovascular Health at Mount Sinai Heart, New York, NY, USA

© Springer International Publishing AG 2018   149
M.M. Berger (ed.), *Critical Care Nutrition Therapy for Non-nutritionists*, https://doi.org/10.1007/978-3-319-58652-6_12

Critical illness can be considered within a four-stage model as acute (days 0–3), prolonged (after day 3 until CCI), CCI (after tracheostomy), and recovery. At approximately day 3 following the acute insult, hypothalamic-pituitary function is dampened, affecting all the major hypothalamic-anterior pituitary hormone axes. As the course progresses, hypercatabolism, inflammation, immobilization, and malnutrition manifest as a CCI syndrome [2, 3].

The initial condition leading to critical illness becomes less important as stereotypical CCI pathophysiology develops. Supportive care that targets metabolic and nutritional needs is associated with reductions in rates of sepsis by 50%, the need for surgery by 55%, and pressure ulcers by 55%, as well as a diminished number of overall complications and a modest improvement post-CCI quality of life [2, 4, 5]. Though hospital readmission rate is unchanged, specialized care provided during CCI has been shown to reduce length of stay during hospital readmission by 4 days [6].

12.2   Malnutrition, Cachexia, and Underfeeding

Malnutrition can be defined as unhealthy networked interactions of dietary factors with metabolism at molecular, biochemical, and physiological scales resulting in abnormal body composition, functional state, and adverse clinical outcomes [7]. Cachexia, characterized by unintentional loss of body mass with muscle wasting, anasarca, and variable adiposity, is highly prevalent among patients with CCI [2].

A number of published screening tools may be used to estimate the risk of malnutrition in CCI [8]. Overall, malnutrition is reported in 43–51% of patients with critical illness and in over 90% of critically ill patients above the age of 70 [2, 9, 10]. Underfeeding is observed in approximately 60–70% of critically ill patients [5].

Feeding should be initiated within 24–48 h of intensive care unit (ICU) admission, though American guidelines emphasize only enteral nutrition (EN), while European guidelines allow for EN and/or parenteral nutrition (PN) early in critical illness [8, 11]. Institutional practices may vary; nutrition is often delayed or disrupted [5]. As a result of underfeeding and severity of illness, nearly all patients that progress to CCI are at high risk for malnutrition and malnutrition-associated complications [5].

12.3   Hypercatabolism and Autophagy

In CCI, the metabolic response to systemic inflammation in critical illness fails to downregulate, leading to increased catabolism, including proteolysis, lipolysis, and reduced hepatic protein synthesis. Residual muscle weakness is observed for at least 2 years following critical illness. Hyperglycemia is commonly observed, along with increased circulating triglycerides and free fatty acids, due to increased lipolysis and reduced utilization.

Enhanced autophagy, a process by which individual cells consume internal organelles as a means of "housekeeping," has been proposed as a contributor to the CCI syndrome [12]. Autophagy is induced by oxidative stress, starvation, and glucagon and is inhibited by insulin and nutrition provision. The complete role of autophagy during critical illness remains unclear: this process may serve to promote protein recycling, limit cellular infection, and mitigate inflammation but may also be responsible for organ dysfunction and loss of lean tissues that are prevalent in CCI [12].

12.4   Nutritional Intervention

With the exception of those few that can feed themselves, nearly all patients that have progressed to CCI should be given nutrition support in the form of EN or PN [8]. These methods are not exclusionary; it is not uncommon for CCI patients to require combined EN and PN in order to meet their nutritional needs [13].

Nutritional assessment of patients with CCI should include a general workup of organ function (renal, hepatic, etc.) and assessment for weight loss, edema, and muscle wasting. Serum testing for micronutrient deficiency is often unnecessary, except in individual cases in which specific deficiencies are suspected. Measurement of serum proteins (e.g., prealbumin, albumin) is discouraged since these levels reflect severity of illness during CCI rather than protein stores [8].

To identify targets, the accurate assessment of evolving energy requirements can be made with the use of indirect calorimetry (IC). Measurement of IC is performed with devices that connect directly to the respiratory circuit of the mechanical ventilator [14]. Continual reassessment is ideal to address changing metabolic targets during CCI. When IC is not available, one of the many published equations for the estimation of daily calorie requirements should be implemented, though their accuracy in CCI has not been established [15].

Adequate protein should be provided, which may be given as 1.0–1.5 g protein/kg body weight daily and at higher rates (1.5–2.5 g/kg) in CCI patients receiving hemodialysis [8, 11]. Measurement of 24 h urine urea nitrogen at 1–2 week intervals can verify the patient's protein needs during CCI [8].

Case identification and aggressive nutrition support are ideal early in the course of critical care. The provision of "extra" calories or protein to malnourished CCI patients does not compensate for prior deficits and places the patient at risk for hyperglycemia, uremia, and hepatosteatosis. Anabolic processes that would confer weight regain are disrupted in CCI and are only employed gradually during the recovery phase. A strategy of targeted metabolic support to meet daily needs in CCI prevents further losses.

12.5   Implementation of EN

The use of EN as a means of nutrition support requires the placement of a feeding tube. Due to expected prolonged use and potential for epithelial erosion, nasally inserted feeding

TABLE 12.1 Specialized enteral tube feed formulas and indications [8]

Type of enteral formula	Nutritional characterization	Clinical indications
Semi-elemental	Partially hydrolyzed protein	Clinical suspicion of malabsorption, intestinal ischemia, prolonged diarrhea
Elemental	Amino acids and short peptides	Clinical suspicion of malabsorption, intestinal ischemia, prolonged diarrhea
High-protein Renal formula	Concentrated, low potassium, low phosphorus	Volume overload, renal insufficiency, hyperkalemia, hyperphosphatemia
Diabetes formula[a]	Lower glucose	Hyperglycemia despite insulin

[a]It should be noted that several feed formulas that are not specifically designated "diabetes" formulas are available that also have low glucose content and would be suitable to administer in patients with hyperglycemia. These include several semi-elemental formulas

tubes should be avoided or replaced with gastric tubes or jejunal tubes.

The choice of tube feed formula should be made individually. In most instances, standard tube feeds represent the most cost-effective approach for adequate nutrition among CCI patients. Specialized feed formulas are available for selective use (Table 12.1) [2, 8].

12.6 Implementation of PN

PN should be considered among CCI patients who do not receive adequate nutrition with the use of EN, including either patients with insufficient EN provision or intolerant of any EN, both usually occurring in cases of gastrointestinal tract dysfunction but also in cases where EN is refused or otherwise contraindicated. PN given either via a central catheter or via a peripheral catheter can potentially provide sufficient calories, protein, lipid, and micronutrients.

Principal risks of PN include line infections at rates of 1.5 infections per 1000 catheter days [16], hepatic dysfunction as both hepatosteatosis and cholestasis, hyperglycemia, volume overload, and other electrolyte derangements. The consideration for PN use should weigh these risks against potential nutritional benefits for the individual patient. Consequently, the timing for initiation of PN in critical illness remains controversial.

The largest published randomized trial compared the use of PN upon arrival to the ICU with PN supplementation starting on ICU day 7 in addition to EN in all patients [17]. Results in the early PN group demonstrated increased length of ICU stay by 1 day, increased length of hospitalization, and higher rates of infections, though lower rates of hypoglycemia [17]. However, only 30% of patients enrolled in this trial remained critically ill for longer than 7 days, and only 6% progressed to CCI. Additionally, all patients enrolled in this trial received a 20% dextrose infusion during the first 2 days of critical illness, which differs from routine ICU practices and recommendations [8, 11].

Another trial that compared provision of PN to supplement EN on ICU days 4 through 8 demonstrated no difference in mortality or length of stay with this intervention compared to the group that received EN alone [13]. Only patients who were expected to remain in the ICU for 5 days or greater were enrolled. Results demonstrate an approximate 30% decrease in rate of nosocomial infections with early PN use, suggesting a potential benefit that may carry over to CCI.

A third study that also compared supplemental PN and EN to standard EN feeding early in critical illness demonstrated no difference in length of stay, mortality, or infection rates [4]. However, the early PN group required mechanical ventilation for approximately 1 day less than the control group, potentially mitigating progression to CCI (though rates of tracheostomy are not reported). Additionally, the early PN group demonstrated less muscle and fat loss, and these improvements appeared to increase throughout the duration of ICU stay, extending through CCI. A small improvement in quality of life after hospital discharge was also noted in the early PN group.

All of these trials evaluated the use of PN during the early stages of critical illness and may suggest metabolic benefits that are retained in CCI. By study design, the entire subset of patients that progressed to CCI within these studies was given PN to supplement insufficient EN intake, including both in the control and experimental arms. One major set of published guidelines favors the use of PN to supplement insufficient EN intake (<60% target calories) after 7–10 days of critical illness [8], while another major set of published guidelines recommends PN supplementation after 2 days of critical illness [11]. By all of these accounts, patients that have progressed to CCI should receive PN either as the sole nutritional source or as a supplement to EN in order to provide complete nutritional support.

12.7   Micronutrient Deficiency

Within these modes of feeding, patients who receive at least 1400 kcal daily of EN or those who receive PN containing multivitamins and trace elements are given amounts of micronutrients to meet average daily requirements. However, increased utilization often renders CCI patients depleted in antioxidant vitamin stores, including vitamins A, C, E, and selenium. Presently, there is insufficient clinical evidence to support supplementation with antioxidants in CCI patients [8]. Randomized trials evaluating antioxidant use in critical illness generally show no significant improvements in clinical outcomes, and within these trials, only a subset of study participants progress to CCI [18, 19].

There is also insufficient evidence to support supplementation with immune-modulating nutritional components such as glutamine, arginine, or nucleic acids [8]. Supplementation with L-carnitine at 1–4 g/day can mitigate deficiency of this micronutrient that commonly develops in CCI and may diminish the risk of hepatosteatosis in patients receiving PN [20].

Vitamin D insufficiency is reported in 91–97% of CCI patients [21]. Serum vitamin D levels have been inversely correlated to ICU outcome; however, clinical evidence to support benefits of supplementation is lacking. One small randomized trial demonstrated vitamin D supplementation in CCI patients did not affect the high rate of bone turnover [22]. Another randomized trial of 25 ICU patients showed vitamin D supplementation improved parathyroid-calcium metabolism, but had no effect on mortality or on length of stay [23].

Iron deficiency should be suspected in patients that require prolonged courses of PN. Iron is typically not included within PN formulations as it may disrupt the lipid emulsification. Oral or parenteral iron supplementation (e.g., iron sucrose 100 mg every 72 h for 15 days) can restore normal levels (Table 12.2).

Copper and zinc deficiencies have been reported in patients receiving continuous renal replacement therapy [24]. Supplementation within this subset of CCI patients may be warranted. Since both copper and zinc compete for absorption and excretion, both should be supplemented concurrently to avoid inducing deficiencies.

TABLE 12.2 Suggested testing schedule

Clinical test	Frequency
Weight	On admission, subsequently every 5–7 days
Indirect calorimetry	On ICU day 2–4, subsequently every 7–14 days
Electrolytes, hepatic function tests, blood urea nitrogen	Every 1–3 days while receiving PN
Serum or plasma glucose	As clinically indicated
Iron, soluble transferrin receptors	After 2–4 weeks of PN as sole nutrition source
Copper, zinc	After 4 weeks of continuous renal replacement

12.8   Endocrine Function and Bone Metabolism

One hallmark of CCI is dampened hypothalamic-pituitary function leading to reduced growth hormone, thyrotropin and thyroid hormone levels, testosterone and estrogens, and potential for reduced cortisol. Of these deficiencies, glucocorticoid replacement should be administered in the case of adrenal insufficiency [25]. Otherwise, hormonal treatment is generally not recommended.

Growth hormone replacement leads to increased mortality and should be avoided [26]. There is insufficient evidence to recommend treatment of non-thyroidal illness with thyroid hormone replacement; current guidelines recommend against this practice [27]. Several small trials suggest improvement in muscle mass with testosterone replacement among male CCI patients. Oxandrolone, a less potent androgen, may also be considered in hypogonadal CCI patients. However, larger trials to evaluate the safety of either treatment have not been conducted [28].

Bone resorption is increased in CCI by systemic inflammation, diminished hypothalamic activity, disuse, and prolonged immobilization [21]. The use of pamidronate in CCI to prevent bone resorption is associated with a reduction in 1-year mortality [29]. A trial of ibandronate, a less potent bisphosphonate, failed to show efficacy [30]. The highly potent anti-resorptive agent denosumab has great potential for benefit in this population, though further study is needed [21].

12.9   Conclusion

CCI represents an extreme, highly catabolic condition in which patients are at heightened risk for malnutrition. Assessment of nutritional needs and provision of nutrition support in the form of EN, EN supplemented by PN, or PN alone remain an important part in the care of all patients that progress to CCI. Published trials that evaluate the use of supplemental PN given early in a patient's ICU course suggest several benefits that become apparent during CCI. Common micronutrient deficiencies that develop in CCI should be addressed. Treatment of increased bone resorption in CCI may also be considered.

References

1. Girard K, Raffin TA. The chronically critically ill: to save or let die? Respir Care. 1985;30(5):339–47.
2. Schulman RC, Mechanick JI. Metabolic and nutrition support in the chronic critical illness syndrome. Respir Care. 2012;57(6):958–77. discussion 977–58.
3. Evans AS, Hosseinian L, Mohabir T, Kurtis S, Mechanick JI. Nutrition and the cardiac surgery intensive care unit patient — an update. J Cardiothorac Vasc Anesth. 2015;29(4):1044–50.
4. Doig GS, Simpson F, Sweetman EA, Finfer SR, Cooper DJ, Heighes PT, Davies AR, O'Leary M, Solano T, Peake S. Early parenteral nutrition in critically ill patients with short-term relative contraindications to early enteral nutrition: a randomized controlled trial. JAMA. 2013;309(20):2130–8.
5. Dvir D, Cohen J, Singer P. Computerized energy balance and complications in critically ill patients: an observational study. Clin Nutr. 2006;25(1):37–44.
6. Daly BJ, Douglas SL, Kelley CG, O'Toole E, Montenegro H. Trial of a disease management program to reduce hospital readmissions of the chronically critically ill. Chest. 2005;128(2):507–17.
7. Mechanick JI, Via MA, Zhao SZ, editors. Molecular nutrition. Washington, DC: Endocrine Press; 2015.
8. McClave SA, Taylor BE, Martindale RG, Warren MM, Johnson DR, Braunschweig C, McCarthy MS, Davanos E, Rice TW, Cresci GA, et al. Guidelines for the provision and assessment of nutrition support therapy in the adult critically ill patient: Society of Critical Care Medicine (SCCM) and American Society for Parenteral and Enteral Nutrition (A.S.P.E.N.). JPEN J Parenter Enteral Nutr. 2016;40(2):159–211.
9. Sanchez-Rodriguez D, Marco E, Ronquillo-Moreno N, Miralles R, Vazquez-Ibar O, Escalada F, Muniesa JM. Prevalence of malnutrition and sarcopenia in a post-acute care geriatric unit: applying the new ESPEN definition and EWGSOP criteria. Clin Nutr. 2017;36(5):1339–44.

10. Mogensen KM, Robinson MK, Casey JD, Gunasekera NS, Moromizato T, Rawn JD, Christopher KB. Nutritional status and mortality in the critically ill. Crit Care Med. 2015;43(12):2605–15.
11. Singer P, Berger MM, Van den Berghe G, Biolo G, Calder P, Forbes A, Griffiths R, Kreyman G, Leverve X, Pichard C, et al. ESPEN guidelines on parenteral nutrition: intensive care. Clin Nutr. 2009;28(4):387–400.
12. McClave SA, Weijs PJ. Preservation of autophagy should not direct nutritional therapy. Curr Opin Clin Nutr Metab Care. 2015;18(2):155–61.
13. Heidegger CP, Berger MM, Graf S, Zingg W, Darmon P, Costanza MC, Thibault R, Pichard C. Optimisation of energy provision with supplemental parenteral nutrition in critically ill patients: a randomised controlled clinical trial. Lancet. 2013;381(9864):385–93.
14. Oshima T, Berger MM, De Waele E, Guttormsen AB, Heidegger CP, Hiesmayr M, Singer P, Wernerman J, Pichard C. Indirect calorimetry in nutritional therapy. A position paper by the ICALIC Study Group. Clin Nutr. 2017;36(3):651–62.
15. Kruizenga HM, Hofsteenge GH, Weijs PJ. Predicting resting energy expenditure in underweight, normal weight, overweight, and obese adult hospital patients. Nutr Metab (Lond). 2016;13:85.
16. Dyson JK, Thompson N. Adult parenteral nutrition in the North of England: a region-wide audit. BMJ Open. 2017;7(1):e012663.
17. Casaer MP, Mesotten D, Hermans G, Wouters PJ, Schetz M, Meyfroidt G, Van Cromphaut S, Ingels C, Meersseman P, Muller J, et al. Early versus late parenteral nutrition in critically ill adults. N Engl J Med. 2011;365(6):506–17.
18. Koekkoek WA, van Zanten AR. Antioxidant vitamins and trace elements in critical illness. Nutr Clin Pract. 2016;31(4):457–74.
19. Berger MM, Soguel L, Shenkin A, Revelly JP, Pinget C, Baines M, Chiolero RL. Influence of early antioxidant supplements on clinical evolution and organ function in critically ill cardiac surgery, major trauma, and subarachnoid hemorrhage patients. Crit Care. 2008;12(4):R101.
20. Bonafe L, Berger MM, Que YA, Mechanick JI. Carnitine deficiency in chronic critical illness. Curr Opin Clin Nutr Metab Care. 2014;17(2):200–9.
21. Via MA, Gallagher EJ, Mechanick JI. Bone physiology and therapeutics in chronic critical illness. Ann N Y Acad Sci. 2010;1211:85–94.

22. Van den Berghe G, Van Roosbroeck D, Vanhove P, Wouters PJ, De Pourcq L, Bouillon R. Bone turnover in prolonged critical illness: effect of vitamin D. J Clin Endocrinol Metab. 2003;88(10):4623–32.
23. Amrein K, Sourij H, Wagner G, Holl A, Pieber TR, Smolle KH, Stojakovic T, Schnedl C, Dobnig H. Short-term effects of high-dose oral vitamin D3 in critically ill vitamin D deficient patients: a randomized, double-blind, placebo-controlled pilot study. Crit Care. 2011;15(2):R104.
24. Ben-Hamouda N, Charriere M, Voirol P, Berger MM. Massive copper and selenium losses cause life-threatening deficiencies during prolonged continuous renal replacement. Nutrition. 2017;34:71–5.
25. Annane D, Bellissant E, Bollaert PE, Briegel J, Confalonieri M, De Gaudio R, Keh D, Kupfer Y, Oppert M, Meduri GU. Corticosteroids in the treatment of severe sepsis and septic shock in adults: a systematic review. JAMA. 2009;301(22):2362–75.
26. Takala J, Ruokonen E, Webster NR, Nielsen MS, Zandstra DF, Vundelinckx G, Hinds CJ. Increased mortality associated with growth hormone treatment in critically ill adults. N Engl J Med. 1999;341(11):785–92.
27. Garber JR, Cobin RH, Gharib H, Hennessey JV, Klein I, Mechanick JI, Pessah-Pollack R, Singer PA, Woeber KA. Clinical practice guidelines for hypothyroidism in adults: cosponsored by the American Association of Clinical Endocrinologists and the American Thyroid Association. Endocr Pract. 2012;18(6):988–1028.
28. Nierman DM, Mechanick JI. Hypotestosteronemia in chronically critically ill men. Crit Care Med. 1999;27(11):2418–21.
29. Schulman RC, Moshier EL, Rho L, Casey MF, Godbold JH, Zaidi M, Mechanick JI. Intravenous pamidronate is associated with reduced mortality in patients with chronic critical illness. Endocr Pract. 2016;22(7):799–808.
30. Via MA, Potenza MV, Hollander J, Liu X, Peng Y, Li J, Sun L, Zaidi M, Mechanick JI. Intravenous ibandronate acutely reduces bone hyperresorption in chronic critical illness. J Intensive Care Med. 2012;27(5):312–8.

Chapter 13
Practical Aspects of Nutrition

Mélanie Charrière and Mette M. Berger

The main purpose of nutritional support is to prevent malnutrition and its associated complications [1]. This objective will be achieved by providing the appropriate doses of macro- and micronutrients (1) to meet the needs of the individual patient by either enteral or parenteral route and (2) to prevent complications associated with nutritional support, through an optimised feed delivery technique [2]. Whatever the route, feeding protocol must but created integrating local possibilities describing the respective tasks of nurses, dieticians and doctors.

M. Charrière, R.D.* • M.M. Berger, M.D., Ph.D. (✉)
*Service of Endocrinology, Diabetes and Metabolism,
University Hospital CHUV, Lausanne, Switzerland

Service of Intensive Care Medicine and Burns,
University Hospital CHUV, Lausanne, Switzerland
e-mail: Mette.Berger@chuv.ch

© Springer International Publishing AG 2018   161
M.M. Berger (ed.), *Critical Care Nutrition Therapy
for Non-nutritionists*, https://doi.org/10.1007/978-3-319-58652-6_13

13.1   Enteral Nutrition

The enteral nutrition (EN) is the first choice, because of its positive effects on the gut (motility preservation, immune function, intestinal mucosal atrophy and bacterial translocation prevention) [3].

13.1.1   Indications and Contraindications

Patients with a functioning gut should receive enteral feeding, if they are unable to eat or to cover 70% of their nutritional needs by the oral route within the next 3 days. In case of partial oral feeding, the 30–40% of the needs may be covered with oral nutrition supplements (ONS).

The absolute contraindications to EN are ileus, mechanical obstruction, active gastrointestinal haemorrhage and severe haemodynamic instability [2].

13.1.2   Timing

Enteral feeding should be started early, within the first 24–48 h following admission, to facilitate diet tolerance and take the advantage of EN benefits (ESICM guidelines 2017 [4]).

EN should be delayed beyond 48 h in uncontrolled shock, uncontrolled hypoxaemia and acidosis, uncontrolled upper gastrointestinal bleeding, gastric aspirate >500 mL/6 h, bowel ischaemia, bowel obstruction, abdominal compartment syndrome and high-output fistula without distal feeding access [4].

13.1.3   Access and Technique

Nasogastric tube is the most common and simple access. Blind insertion on bedside can be done by a trained nurse. A polyurethane fine-bore tube is more comfortable for the patient. Before initiating enteral feeding, it is important to confirm nasogastric tube position on a chest X-ray, because clinical control by air insufflation is frequently misleading. Once the tube is in place, remove any guidewire, secure it carefully, and document tube insertion in the patient's follow-up chart. Try to avoid any compression points, for example, at the nose, which could lead to skin necrosis.

Postpyloric tubes, although efficient on occasions in the presence of persistent high gastric residual volumes, do not offer a systematic advantage over gastric tubes as shown by a randomised trial to either route [5]: nasojejunal tubes did not increase energy delivery and did not reduce the frequency of pneumonia.

Percutaneous endoscopic gastrostomy (PEG), with jejunal tube or surgical access (gastrostomy, jejunostomy) should be considered if the patient will be requiring long term EN support after the critical care.

Patient position is a major issue: the head of the bed should always be in a 30–45° tilt position.

In the ICU setting, the continuous administration of EN is preferred to bolus feeding to prevent regurgitation and important variations in glycaemia and insulin requirements. A dedicated pump is required to guarantee target energy intake and optimise gastric tolerance.

EN should be initiated at a rate of 20–30 mL/h and regularly increased according to bowel tolerance assessed by gastric residual volumes (GRV) that are best measured every 12 h during the first 72 h of EN initiation, particularly in surgical patients. More frequent GRV measurement is counterproductive as it only achieves a reduction of feed delivery. Figure 13.1 shows a reasonable progression modus over 3 days.

13.1.4   Feeding Products

Polymeric formulas are appropriate for the majority of patients. They are lactose-free and gluten-free. Nutrients are not hydrolysed, resulting in a moderate osmolality close to physiological levels (300–350 mOsmol/L) [6]. Several formulas are available (high or low protein, semi-elemental,

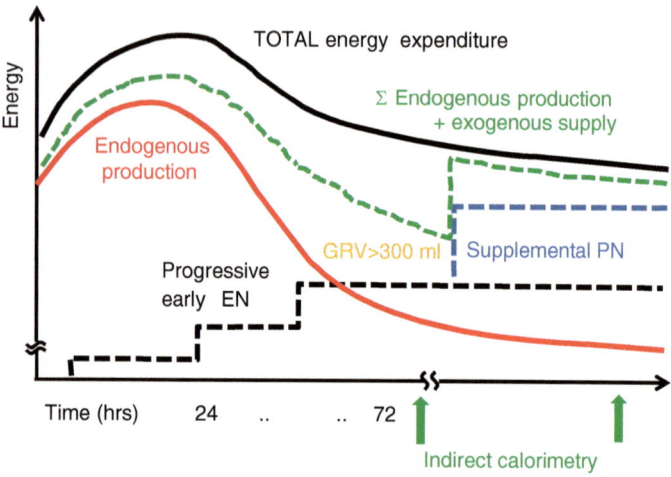

FIGURE 13.1 Conceptual description of feeding progression, the same feeding progression applies whatever the route of feeding (Reproduced with permission from Oshima T, Berger MM, De Waele E, et al. Indirect calorimetry in nutritional therapy. A position paper by the ICALIC Study Group. Clin Nutr. 2017;36:651–62)

disease specific, high fat, diabetes, etc.). The presence of multiple different products in the ICU results in confusion, which in turn leads to non-using any: it is more efficient including for the pharmacy to choose one standard product—the niche indications to other products should occur under the supervision of a trained ICU dietician.

1. *Energy*: the formulas should be modestly hypercaloric, i.e. 1.3–1.5 kcal/mL, to provide energy and protein and meet targets without compromising fluid control. The more energy dense formulas favour gastric retention.
2. *Proteins*: to provide 1.2–1.5 g/kg/day and simultaneously respect the target energy of 20–25 kcal/kg, the enteral formula should contain at least 25% of energy as proteins. New whey-containing products are coming on the market that may enable solving this conundrum.
3. *Carbohydrates*: there is a wide variation in the content. Nevertheless, considering the substrate requirements, 50–55% of total energy should be provided under that form.

4. *Lipids*: many solutions have high fat content in order to increase energy content and are frequently used in muco-viscidosis, but have no proven benefit in critical illness. The amount of lipid energy should be monitored particularly in case of propofol sedation which adds large amounts of fat [7]. EN products with maximum 35% of energy as fat should be preferred.

5. *Fibres*: while long debated, evidence slowly accumulates in favour of their inclusion from the beginning of nutritional support. Insoluble fibres increase faecal mass by entrapping water. Soluble fibres are well fermented by colonic anaerobic microflora and provide substrates, which maintain the structure and function of the colon [6]. A dose of 15–20 g/day seems clinically adequate.

6. *Electrolytes and micronutrients*: with the delivery of 1500 kcal/day, the requirements are usually met (Recommendes daily intake = RDI). However, in the ICU, increased nutritional requirements and/or loss of specific nutrients must be considered, and additional micronutrient is frequently required.

Good clinical and hygiene practices prevent infections and diarrhoea. Hand disinfection procedures should be systematic before manipulating feeding tubes and formulas, because of the risk of bacterial colonisation. EN infusion sets should be changed every 24 h. Feeds should not be administrated for more than 24 h. Avoiding any manipulation such as mixing feeds in a single bag is recommended.

13.1.5   Complications

The figure 13.2 summarizes common complications of artificial nutritional support. Hereafter we discuss three of them.

Underfeeding: actual nutrient delivery must be checked every day, especially because feeding interruptions frequently occur in the ICU for several reasons, such as patient transport for investigations or preparation for procedures. In the case of EN interruption, the feeding rate may be raised transiently, if the patient tolerates it, in order to meet the daily energy

Complications	Preventive and/or therapeutic actions
Gastric residual volume >300 ml	1. Administer prokinetic drugs 2. Use postpyloric feeding tube 3. Use supplemental PN
Bronchoaspiration	Elevate patient's head to at least 30° (ideal 45°)
Tube obstruction	− Prevent with regular 20 ml water flush − Use good practices when delivering medication through feeding tube
Aspiration pneumonia due to tube displacement	Check tube position: − Before administering food and/or medications; − If vomiting or coughing; − If the visible portion of the tube seems longer than previously measured (clue for displacement)
Underfeeding	− Verify daily that patient is receiving the amount of nutrients that were prescribed − If not, consider supplemental PN after 3 days [9]
Constipation	− Check for hydration − Use fibres supplementation − Give prokinetic drugs
Diarrhoea	− Prevent constipation early and gently − Optimize hygiene practices − Give fibres, osmolar feeding <300 mOsm − Control infusion rate − Use supplemental PN [11]

FIGURE 13.2 Complications of enteral nutrition

target [8]. If we can deliver at least 60% of the energy target with enteral feeding, a supplemental PN (parenteral nutrition) should be initiated to cover the needs [9].

Constipation occurs in 70% of patients on EN [10]. Prevention is best realised by the use of polyethylene glycols (macrogol) from the start.

Diarrhoea: the most frequent causes of diarrhoea are antibiotics. But it occurs in 14% of patients and is associated with EN > 60% of energy target [11] and can cause or accentuate malnutrition.

13.1.6   Specific Monitoring

Daily real feed delivery enables detection of trouble and daily and cumulated energy balance calculation (target minus delivery), as well as protein target achievement.

Tube position should be checked daily, either on a chest X-ray as required by respiratory treatment, by air insufflation or at least by checking the distance marks at the nostril.

Gastric residual volume should be checked every 12 h upon initiation of EN until they remain <100 mL or in general for the first 3 days of EN.

Clinical observation: consider oedema that may hide the loss of lean body mass.

13.2   Parenteral Nutrition

Total parenteral nutrition (PN) is a way of supplying all the nutritional needs of the body by bypassing the digestive system and dripping nutrient solution directly into a vein. This implies two major constraints: strict aseptic technique and a central venous catheter. It also includes selecting the appropriate patients, the most appropriate access, the choice of the nutrient solution, the adapted monitoring and the awareness about the stability concerns in case of additions.

PN was until recently considered to cause worse outcomes than EN. This was indeed the case in the 1980s–1990s for mainly three reasons: (1) as PN had been developed to treat malnutrition in the 1970s, it frequently resulted in overfeeding with its deleterious effects (PN was named hyperalimentation); (2) with overfeeding, hyperglycaemia was not controlled, favouring infectious complications; (3) the PN solutions were less balanced regarding fat and amino acid composition than the EN solutions. With modern solutions and moderate energy targets, the outcomes of EN and PN are similar, as demonstrated by randomised trials [12]. PN may even generate an outcome benefit when EN is temporarily contraindicated [13] or insufficient [9], by the prevention of underfeeding and its consequences.

13.2.1   Indications

The fundamental indication to total PN is intestinal failure, which can be short, medium or long term, sometimes years. A partial gut failure may be an indication to a combined feeding regimen, with variable amounts of the needs being supplied by PN.

13.2.2   Timing

The timing of PN initiation is a source of controversy among the nutrition societies. The European position is to consider that in critical care patients, it should be considered in case of EN failure from day 4 and might be indicated from the first ICU day, if some conditions are fulfilled (Table 13.1 and Fig. 13.1).

TABLE 13.1 Timing of PN initiation according to the European concept

Timing	Indication—comment
Admission days 1–2	PN initiated before admission to the ICU due to contraindication to enteral feeding Malnutrition upon admission
Days 3–4	Enteral nutrition not covering 60% of energy targets ESPEN guidelines [19]
Later	Whenever the intestinal tract fails ASPEN guidelines from day 7 [20]

13.2.3   Access

The ICU patient is frequently equipped with multi-lumen central venous lines for therapeutic reasons. In case of PN, one lumen should be dedicated to the PN solution to reduce the number of manipulations and associated infectious risks.

In case a new line is required, the site associated with the least infectious risks is the subclavian site: it is followed by the jugular site and thereafter by the femoral site. Other advantages of the subclavian site are to be easiest to nurse and more comfortable for the patient. Under circumstances, a peripherally inserted catheter (PIC line) might be an alternative, placed in the cephalic, basilic or brachial veins.

Whenever a new line is inserted, the procedure should be performed under strict surgical aseptic conditions. The verification of the distal position of the catheter on an X-ray belongs to standard care: the tip should lie within the superior vena cava above the junction with the right atrium.

Peripheral access is an unusual option in the ICU (Fig. 13.3), due to the frequent availability of a central line and to the necessity to change the peripheral catheters due to the rapidly (3–4 days) occurring chemical phlebitis.

13.2.4   Nutrients

As the entire nutritional, fluid and electrolyte requirements should be covered, the provision of a balanced and complete blend of macronutrients (carbohydrates, amino acids, lipids), micronutrients (trace elements and vitamins) and electrolytes is required. For tolerance reasons (direct injection into the circulating compartment), the nutrients are provided in molecular form, which is very different from enteral feeds. It results in hyperosmolar solutions (Table 13.2):

Site	Advantages	Disadvantages
Peripheral	– Lower osmolality than central (650–850 mmol/l) – Rescue therapy in presence of extensive thrombotic complications – Can be used a supplemental PN to cover 500–600 kcal/day are required and enteral tube is unavailable	– Limited concentration of energy and nutrients (lipids dominate) – Limited amino acid provision – Requires large volumes of fluid for full feeing (2.5–3 L/dh) – Risk of hypervolemia (detrimental in case of cardiac failure) – Requires a rich peripheral venous pool – Required trace elements and vitamins are poorly tolerated causing phlebitis
Central	– Concentrated nutrients (1.08–1.4 kcal/ml), limiting the fluid overload – Enables providing 1.1–1.2 g/kg/d of amino acids – Compounding is possible	– Hyperosmolar (1400–2000 mosm/l) – Industrial solutions usually provide limited amounts of amino acids

FIGURE 13.3 Comparison of peripheral versus central PN in ICU patients

1. *Carbohydrates* are supplied as glucose, in more or less concentrated forms (40–70%).
2. *Proteins* are provided as amino acids, the bricks of proteins. The crystalline 8–15% amino acid solutions have until now always been incomplete regarding the provision of all amino acids: glutamine, which is a conditionally essential amino acid during critical illness, is particularly missing [14, 15]. Of note, for chemical reasons, when providing 1 g of amino acids, one should be aware that it contains about 17% less nitrogen than 1 g of protein: a molecule of water is released when a peptide bond is formed.
3. *Lipids* are provided as triglycerides, composed of a glycerol backbone on which three fatty acids (FA) are attached. The FA are of different types: actual fat emulsions provide a balanced blend of medium chain triglycerides (MCT), n-3, n-6 and n-9 FA. For a comprehensive discussion, see review by Calder [16].
4. *Electrolytes*: industrial ready to use solutions contain a blend of electrolytes in moderate amounts.

TABLE 13.2 Comparison of enteral and parenteral feeding solutions

Substrate	Enteral nutrients	Parenteral solutions
Physical presentation	All-in-one container	Triple-chamber bags ready to mix
Carbohydrates	Maltodextrins	Glucose
Proteins	Full blend of polymeric proteins, including glutamine, 8%	Amino acids, incomplete blend, in particular the absence of glutamine
Lipids	Mix of fatty acids with variable proportions of MCT, n-6, n-9 and n-3 fatty acids	Fatty acids (FA): Two recent products offer a mixture of four FA (MCT, n-3, n-6, n-9)
Electrolytes	Covers normal requirements of Na, K, P, Ca and Mg	Moderate quantities of Na, K, Mg, Ca and P Optional: no electrolytes in the bag—frequently preferred in the ICU
Micronutrients (trace elements, vitamins)	Recommended daily intakes for 1500 kcal	None

5. *Micronutrients*: for stability reasons, the PN solutions contain no micronutrients. To prevent incomplete feeding, a separate administration of daily doses of trace elements and vitamins is required [17]. The micronutrients may be added to the PN solution on the day of administration, keeping in mind that vitamin C needs light protection and nearly disappears after 3–4 h of daylight exposure.

13.2.5 Ready to Use Industrial Bags

Separate substrate infusion is no more recommended. Triple-chamber bags are available from several companies. This presentation provides a longer storage time, provided trace elements and vitamins are not added to it. Some hospital pharmacies are able to realise compounding of PN solutions, with individually adapted substrate composition: this enables the production of PN with lower quantities of fat and higher amounts of amino acids, including glutamine.

13.2.6   Administration of PN

- *Progression of feeding*: like EN, PN should be progressed stepwise to target over 48–72 h, starting at a rate of about 20 mL/h. Depending on the PN solution concentration, this corresponds to 15–20 kcal/h. It should be increased according to glucose tolerance every 12 h, to enable adaptation of the insulin secretion and provision. In case of combined feeding, a similar progression to target applies. This progression limits the risk of refeeding syndrome [18].
- *Perfusions*: pumps are required for continuous 24 h administration. The infusion may be shortened to 8–14 h, generally overnight (called "cyclic PN") during the recovery phase, to enable patient mobilisation. The infusion lines are standard intravenous tubes: the most frequent recommendation is to change them every 3–4 days. A more frequent replacement is costly without demonstrated benefits.
- *Bag duration*: whatever PN bag is used, whenever the bag is opened, it should not be infused for longer than 36 h. The industrial recommendation is a 24 h limitation, but some tolerance is permitted to avoid throwing away bags and substrates.

13.2.7   Specific Monitoring

The recommendations of Chap. 1 particularly apply to PN, with tight monitoring of K and P upon initiation of feeding.

Blood glucose monitoring requires special attention until the prescribed energy target is reached. As the gut is bypassed, the incretions are not stimulated by the food. Hence, the insulinic response is modified, and about 30% more extrinsic insulin is required for the same amount of glucose and the same glycaemic target (6–8 mmol/L).

Liver function tests ought to be determined twice weekly.

13.3 Conclusion

Artificial feeding is a therapy that requires skills, rigour, asepsis, a feeding protocol and a specific technical knowledge. Feeding EN is the first recommendation, but feeding being the aim, its failure summons the use of PN. The latter is a little more complex technically compared to EN but easier for nurses to apply.

References

1. Simpson F, Doig GS. Parenteral vs. enteral nutrition in the critically ill patient: a meta-analysis of trials using the intention to treat principle. Intensive Care Med. 2005;31:12–23.
2. Seron-Arbeloa C, Zamora-Elson M, Labarta-Monzon L, Mallor-Bonet T. Enteral nutrition in critical care. J Clin Med Res. 2013;5:1–11.
3. Gatt M, Reddy BS, MacFie J. Review article: bacterial translocation in the critically ill—evidence and methods of prevention. Aliment Pharmacol Ther. 2007;25:741–57.
4. Reintam Blaser A, Starkopf J, Alhazzani W, Berger MM, Casaer MP, Deane AM, Fruhwald S, Hiesmayr M, Ichai C, Jakob SM, Loudet CI, Malbrain ML, Montejo Gonzalez JC, Paugam-Burtz C, Poeze M, Preiser JC, Singer P, van Zanten AR, De Waele J, Wendon J, Wernerman J, Whitehouse T, Wilmer A, Oudemans-van Straaten HM, Function ESICM Working Group on Gastrointestinal. Early enteral nutrition in critically ill patients: ESICM clinical practice guidelines. Intensive Care Med. 2017;43:380–98.
5. Davies AR, Morrison SS, Bailey MJ, Bellomo R, Cooper DJ, Doig GS, Finfer SR, Heyland DK, Investigators Enteric Study, Anzics Clinical Trials Group. A multicenter, randomized controlled trial comparing early nasojejunal with nasogastric nutrition in critical illness. Crit Care Med. 2012;40:2342–8.

6. Zadak ZM, Nyulasi I, Lochs H, Kent-Smith L, Pirlich M. Commercially prepared diets for enteral nutrition. In: Sobotka L, editor. Basics in clinical nutrition. 2011. 4th ed. pp. 333–43. Prague: Galén.

7. Charrière M, Ridley E, Hastings J, Bianchet O, Scheinkestel C, Berger MM. Propofol sedation substantially increases the caloric and lipid intake in critically ill patients. Nutrition. 2017;42:64–8.

8. Berger MM, Revelly JP, Wasserfallen JB, Schmid A, Bouvry S, Cayeux MC, Musset M, Maravic P, Chiolero RL. Impact of a computerized information system on quality of nutritional support in the ICU. Nutrition. 2006;22:221–9.

9. Heidegger CP, Berger MM, Graf S, Zingg W, Darmon P, Costanza MC, Thibault R, Pichard C. Optimisation of energy provision with supplemental parenteral nutrition in critically ill patients: a randomised controlled clinical trial. Lancet. 2013;381:385–93.

10. Bittencourt AF, Martins JR, Logullo L, Shiroma G, Horie L, Ortolani MC, Silva Mde L, Waitzberg DL. Constipation is more frequent than diarrhea in patients fed exclusively by enteral nutrition: results of an observational study. Nutr Clin Pract. 2012;27:533–9.

11. Thibault R, Graf S, Clerc A, Delieuvin N, Heidegger CP, Pichard C. Diarrhoea in the intensive care unit: respective contribution of feeding and antibiotics. Crit Care. 2013;17:R153.

12. Harvey SE, Parrott F, Harrison DA, Bear DE, Segaran E, Beale R, Bellingan G, Leonard R, Mythen MG, Rowan KM, Investigators Calories Trial. Trial of the route of early nutritional support in critically ill adults—Calories Trial. N Engl J Med. 2014;371:1673–84.

13. Doig GS, Simpson F, Sweetman EA, Finfer SR, Cooper DJ, Heighes PT, Davies AR, O'Leary M, Solano T, Peake S, Early PN, Investigators of the Anzics Clinical Trials Group. Early parenteral nutrition in critically ill patients with short-term relative contraindications to early enteral nutrition: a randomized controlled trial. JAMA. 2013;309:2130–8.

14. Berger MM. The 2013 arvid wretlind lecture: evolving concepts in parenteral nutrition. Clin Nutr. 2014;33:563–70.

15. Stehle P, Ellger B, Kojic D, Feuersenger A, Schneid C, Stover J, Scheiner D, Westphal M. Glutamine dipeptide-supplemented parenteral nutrition improves the clinical outcomes of critically ill patients: a systematic evaluation of randomised controlled trials. Clin Nutr ESPEN. 2017;17:75–85.

16. Calder PC. Lipids for intravenous nutrition in hospitalised adult patients: a multiple choice of options. Proc Nutr Soc. 2013;72:263–76.
17. Singer P, Berger MM, Van den Berghe G, Biolo G, Calder P, Forbes A, Griffiths R, Kreyman G, Leverve X, Pichard C. ESPEN guidelines on parenteral nutrition: intensive care. Clin Nutr. 2009;28:387–400.
18. Doig GS, Simpson F, Heighes PT, Bellomo R, Chesher D, Caterson ID, Reade MC, Harrigan PW, Refeeding Syndrome Trial Investigators Group. Restricted versus continued standard caloric intake during the management of refeeding syndrome in critically ill adults: a randomised, parallel-group, multicentre, single-blind controlled trial. Lancet Respir Med. 2015;3: 943–52.
19. Singer P, Reintam Blaser A, Berger MM, Calder P, Casear M, Hiesmayr M, Mayer K, Montejo JC, Pichard C, Preiser JC, Tepinski P, van Zanten AR. ESPEN guidelines for the critically ill patient. Clinical Nutr. 2018.
20. McClave SA, Taylor BE, Martindale RG, Warren MM, Johnson DR, Braunschweig C, McCarthy MS, Davanos E, Rice TW, Cresci GA, Gervasio JM, Sacks GS, Roberts PR, Compher C, Society of Critical Care Medicine, American Society for Parenteral, Enteral Nutrition. Guidelines for the provision and assessment of nutrition support therapy in the adult critically ill patient: Society of Critical Care Medicine (SCCM) and American Society for Parenteral and Enteral Nutrition (A.S.P.E.N.). JPEN J Parenter Enteral Nutr. 2016;40:159–211.

Index

© Springer International Publishing AG 2018
M.M. Berger (ed.), *Critical Care Nutrition Therapy for
Non-nutritionists*, https://doi.org/10.1007/978-3-319-58652-6